Methanogens - Unique Prokaryotes

Edited by Sevcan Aydin

Published in London, United Kingdom

Methanogens - Unique Prokaryotes
http://dx.doi.org/10.5772/intechopen.1001727
Edited by Sevcan Aydin

Contributors
Fang Yin, Finn O. Gehlert, Jasia Javed, Junlin Ji, Luise Rentz, Muhammad Junaid Ahmad Tariq, Ruth A. Schmitz, Salomeh Chegini, Sameen Meer, Sevcan Aydin, Ume Habiba, Wudi Zhang, Özge Dua Zengin

First published in London, United Kingdom, 2025 by IntechOpen
IntechOpen is the global imprint of INTECHOPEN LIMITED, registered in England and Wales, registration number: 11086078, 167-169 Great Portland Street, London, W1W 5PF, United Kingdom

For EU product safety concerns: IN TECH d.o.o., Prolaz Marije Krucifikse Kozulić 3, 51000 Rijeka, Croatia, info@intechopen.com or visit our website at intechopen.com.

British Library Cataloguing-in-Publication Data
A catalogue record for this book is available from the British Library

Methanogens - Unique Prokaryotes
Edited by Sevcan Aydin
p. cm.
Print ISBN 978-1-83634-155-0
Online ISBN 978-1-83634-154-3
eBook (PDF) ISBN 978-1-83634-156-7

If disposing of this product, please recycle the paper responsibly.

Meet the editor

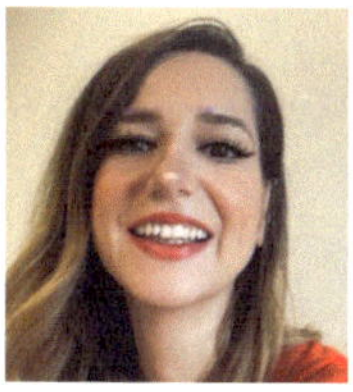

Sevcan Aydin is a Professor in the Biology Department at the Istanbul University in Turkey. She earned her bachelor's degree from the Biology Department of Ege University and a Ph.D. in Environmental Biotechnology from Istanbul Technical University in 2015. Her research focuses on environmental biotechnology, renewable energy, bioremediation, and environmental engineering. With 49 scientific articles published in high-impact journals (SCOPUS citations: 1385, h-index 21), she has supervised 4 doctoral and 8 master's theses. Prof. Aydin teaches biotechnological water treatment, environmental technologies, and bioenergy production. Her expertise centres explicitly on optimizing bioenergy from waste, cost-effective methodologies, and detecting methanogens in anaerobic processes. This multifaceted approach provides valuable insights into the role of microorganisms in environmental dynamics.

Contents

Preface

Methanogens are extraordinary prokaryotes that are indispensable in the Earth's carbon cycle and environmental sustainability. Although they are relatively less studied than other microorganisms, methanogens are crucial in processes such as methane production, carbon recycling, and symbiotic relationships within the gastrointestinal microbiota. *Methanogens – Unique Prokaryotes* is a comprehensive edited volume that explores these fascinating microorganisms, as well as their biological functions, industrial potential, and growing significance across various scientific disciplines.

The first chapter, "Unlocking the Power of Methanogens: Revolutionary Applications in Sustainable Energy and Biotechnology", focuses on the increasing role of methanogens in biotechnology and energy. This chapter examines methanogens' contributions to biogas production, anaerobic digestion processes, and biofuel development. As the global demand for renewable energy continues to rise, methanogens are gaining recognition for their role in reducing greenhouse gas emissions, recycling organic waste, and generating alternative energy sources.

The second chapter, "Pioneering Methanogens: The Architects of Modern Eco-Friendly Renewable Energy Solutions", delves into the transformative power of methanogens in ecological energy production. By emphasizing the biological processes in which methanogens play a key role, this chapter explains how these microorganisms serve as essential components of sustainable energy solutions. The ability of methanogens to efficiently utilize natural resources positions them as promising agents in shaping the future of energy production.

The third chapter, "Genomic Mobility: Transposons in Methanoarchaea", introduces a new perspective on the genetic adaptation processes of methanogens. This chapter explores how mobile genetic elements, such as transposons and plasmids, contribute to methanogens' genetic diversity and evolution. Understanding these mechanisms enhances our knowledge of how methanogens thrive in diverse ecological niches, ranging from the human gut to wetlands and deep-sea environments.

The fourth chapter, "Co-Production of Hydrogen and Methane by Anaerobic Digestion", focuses on the potential roles of methanogens in renewable energy systems. This chapter examines how methanogens can simultaneously produce hydrogen and methane—two energy-rich gases—through anaerobic digestion. The ability of methanogens to facilitate this process offers promising opportunities for developing cleaner, more sustainable, and cost-effective energy production methods.

The final chapter, "The Hidden Influence of Methanogens in the Gut Microbiota", provides a comprehensive understanding of the biological significance of methanogens within the human gut. This chapter explores the complex interactions between methanogens and the gut microbiota, highlighting their role in digestion, immune system regulation, and the gut-brain axis. The potential impact of methanogens on mental health and their association with various neurological disorders present a new frontier in gut microbiome research.

This book is a valuable resource for researchers, professionals, and enthusiasts in microbiology, biotechnology, energy production, and environmental sciences. *Methanogens – Unique Prokaryotes* presents the latest research and technological advancements, emphasizing the interdisciplinary importance of methanogens. This book provides insights into how methanogens contribute to energy production, environmental conservation, and human health by offering a broad perspective on their applications.

This volume results from the collective expertise of many distinguished authors, each contributing to a multidimensional understanding of methanogens. The collaborative efforts of the authors have produced a scientifically rich and practically relevant resource, bridging the gap between fundamental research and industrial applications.

We sincerely thank all authors, editors, and reviewers who contributed to this book. Their dedication and expertise have been instrumental in creating this comprehensive collection of methanogen research. We hope this book will inspire future research and technological advancements, paving the way for further discoveries in the field of methanogen biology.

Dr. Sevcan Aydin
Professor,
Biotechnology Department,
Istanbul University,
Istanbul, Turkey

Chapter 1

Unlocking the Power of Methanogens: Revolutionary Applications in Sustainable Energy and Biotechnology

Salomeh Chegini

Abstract

Methanogens, unique microorganisms within the archaea domain, produce methane as a byproduct of methanogenesis, a crucial process in the global carbon cycle. Thriving in anaerobic environments such as wetlands, landfills, and ruminant guts, these archaea hold tremendous potential for renewable energy and environmental sustainability. This chapter explores the innovative applications of methanogens, including their pivotal role in biogas production, anaerobic digestion, biofuel development, and advanced waste treatment. By leveraging their metabolic versatility and engineering capabilities, methanogens can address pressing challenges in global energy security and carbon neutrality. This chapter provides insights into their metabolic pathways, engineering optimization, and the integration of methanogens into circular economy models and hybrid energy systems. Through case studies, cutting-edge research, and emerging technologies, this work underscores the transformative potential of methanogens in biotechnological and industrial applications. The discussion also highlights challenges, including slow growth rates and environmental sensitivities, while proposing solutions for scaling methanogen-based systems. This overview serves as a valuable resource for researchers, policymakers, and industry stakeholders pursuing innovative methods for biofuel production, environmental management, and carbon capture.

Keywords: methanogens, methanogenesis, anaerobic digestion, biogas production, renewable energy, waste management, carbon capture

1. Introduction

Methanogens, ancient microorganisms from the archaea domain, are uniquely adapted to thrive in oxygen-free environments. Their ability to utilize substrates such as carbon dioxide (CO_2), hydrogen (H_2), and acetate, converting them to methane (CH_4), makes them integral to anaerobic ecosystems and pivotal in sustainable energy innovations [1]. Found in habitats ranging from wetlands to the guts of ruminants, methanogens play a critical role in the global carbon cycle and have gained significant attention for their potential in renewable energy and biotechnology [1].

This chapter explores the role of methanogens in biogas production, biofuel generation, and advanced waste treatment. It discusses innovative strategies, including genetic engineering and co-digestion technologies, which aim to enhance the efficiency of methanogens. Additionally, the chapter addresses challenges such as their sensitivity to environmental fluctuations and their slow metabolic rates, while highlighting technological advancements and potential solutions. The ability of methanogens to convert organic waste into bioenergy positions them as essential players in advancing circular economy models and energy systems globally [1–3].

2. Methanogen metabolism

Methanogens possess distinct cell structures, such as rigid pseudomurein cell walls and specialized coenzymes like coenzyme M, which are essential for methane production. Their ability to survive in extreme conditions, including high salinity and temperature, makes them fascinating subjects for study [4–6].

2.1 Methanogenic pathways

Methanogens utilize three primary metabolic pathways:

Hydrogenotrophic methanogenesis: Uses CO_2 and H_2 to produce methane and water. It is significant in environments rich in hydrogen, such as anaerobic digesters.

Acetoclastic methanogenesis: Converts acetate into methane and CO_2, critical in organic matter degradation. So, this pathway is particularly important in the degradation of organic matter in various ecosystems.

Methylotrophic methanogenesis: This pathway involves the use of methylated compounds, where methanogens convert these substrates into methane. It plays a crucial role in methanogenic communities that inhabit specialized niches [1, 4–7].

3. Methanogens in anaerobic digestion

Anaerobic digestion (AD) is a biological process that dissolves organic matter in the absence of oxygen, producing biogas, primarily composed of methane and carbon dioxide. Methanogens are the essential microorganisms in this process; they are essential for converting volatile fatty acids and hydrogen into methane. The efficiency of anaerobic digestion systems depends on the health and activity of the methanogenic population, which can be influenced by factors such as temperature, pH, and the composition of the substrate. Optimizing conditions for methanogens is crucial for maximizing biogas production and ensuring stable performance in the reactor. The main parameters in the AD process are including [4, 8, 9]:

- *Temperature:* Mesophilic (35–40°C) and thermophilic (50–60°C) ranges optimize methanogen activity.

- *pH:* Neutral conditions (pH ~7.5) enhance methanogenesis.

- *Substrate composition:* Balanced carbon-to-nitrogen ratios improve microbial efficiency.

DOI: http://dx.doi.org/10.5772/intechopen.1009384

3.1 Microbial community dynamics in anaerobic digestion

The anaerobic digestion process involves a synergistic interplay between various microbial communities, each responsible for specific biochemical stages. These microbial groups include hydrolytic bacteria, acidogenic bacteria, acetogenic bacteria, and methanogens. Their interactions and balance are crucial for maintaining system stability and optimizing biogas production [10, 11].

- *Hydrolytic bacteria:* These microbes initiate the digestion process by breaking down complex organic polymers (e.g., carbohydrates, proteins, and lipids) into simpler monomers like sugars, amino acids, and fatty acids. The efficiency of this step is crucial for subsequent microbial activity.

- *Acidogenic bacteria:* These bacteria metabolize the products of hydrolysis, producing volatile fatty acids (VFAs), hydrogen, and carbon dioxide. A balanced VFA production is vital to avoid system inhibition caused by acid accumulation.

- *Acetogenic bacteria:* Acetogens further convert VFAs into acetic acid, hydrogen, and carbon dioxide, serving as precursors for methanogens.

- *Methanogens:* As the ultimate step, methanogens utilize these intermediates to produce methane and carbon dioxide [10, 11].

Figure 1 illustrates the sequential stages of anaerobic digestion, emphasizing the critical role of methanogens in the final methanogenic phase.

The community structure and dynamics in anaerobic digestion (AD) are crucial for the efficient breakdown of organic material into biogas (mainly methane and carbon dioxide).

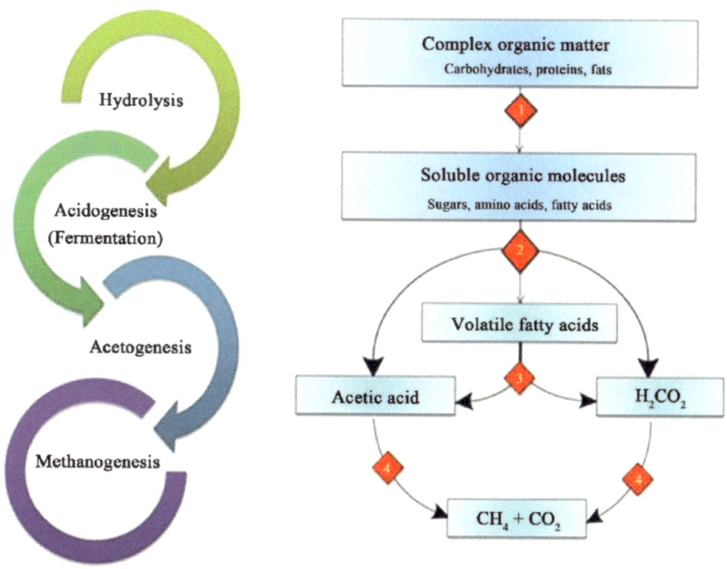

Figure 1.
Anaerobic digestion process [9].

Advanced molecular techniques, such as 16S rRNA gene sequencing and metagenomics, have provided detailed insights into microbial community structure and dynamics [12, 13]:

- *16S rRNA gene sequencing technique* identifies and classifies microorganisms by targeting the highly conserved 16S ribosomal RNA gene, enabling researchers to determine microbial diversity and population structure in an anaerobic digestion system [12, 14].

- *Metagenomics method* provides a more comprehensive view, analyzing the entire genetic material of microbial communities. Metagenomics allows for the identification of functional genes and pathways involved in anaerobic digestion, offering deeper insights into metabolic capabilities and potential interactions among microbes [15].

These methods allow for real-time monitoring and optimization of anaerobic digestion systems by identifying dominant microbial taxa and tracking their responses to operational changes [12, 14, 15].

Also, several environmental and operational factors, such as substrate composition, temperature, pH, and the carbon-to-nitrogen (C/N) ratio, have significant effects on microbial diversity and stability, influencing the process's efficiency and stability. The interaction between these factors shapes the microbial community structure in anaerobic digestion. These microbes work together in distinct phases of the process, from hydrolysis to methanogenesis. Understanding and controlling these factors is essential for optimizing the efficiency and stability of the anaerobic digestion process. Maintaining an appropriate balance ensures that the microbial community remains functional, efficient, and capable of producing biogas at maximum rates. Here is a deeper look into how these factors impact the microbial ecosystem [4, 8, 10, 16]:

3.1.1 pH and volatile fatty acids (VFAs)

Anaerobic digestion generates volatile fatty acids (VFAs) as intermediate products, particularly during the hydrolysis and acidogenesis phases of digestion. If VFAs accumulate to elevated levels, they can lower the pH of the system. A pH drop can be problematic because methanogens (microorganisms that produce methane) are sensitive to pH levels. At low pH, methanogens struggle to function efficiently, which inhibits methane production and can lead to the accumulation of intermediates like VFAs, further disturbing the process. In extreme cases, this can result in process failure methanogenic bacteria thrive at a neutral to slightly alkaline pH, typically around seven. Methanogenic activity, which is the ultimate step of AD, is essential for converting the organic material into methane. A pH drop below 6.5–6.0 can significantly inhibit methanogenesis, causing lower biogas yields or even halting the process altogether [4, 8, 17].

3.1.2 Substrate composition

The type of organic material being digested directly affects the microbial community dynamics. Simple substrates like sugars and proteins are more easily degradable, and the microbial community tends to favor fermentative and acidogenic bacteria in the initial stages. However, more complex materials like lignocellulosic biomass (found in plant materials) are harder to break down. Lignocellulosic materials consist of cellulose, hemicellulose, and lignin, which require the involvement of specialized microbial groups. Municipal solid waste also contains diverse organic fractions, requiring a broad spectrum of enzymatic activities. This necessitates a highly diverse microbial community for efficient degradation [6, 18].

In the case of lignocellulosic substrates, hydrolytic bacteria play a key role in breaking down complex polysaccharides (like cellulose and hemicellulose) into simpler sugars. Acetogenic bacteria then convert these sugars into acetic acid and other VFAs, which serve as substrates for methanogens. The specific types of bacteria that dominate depend on the complexity of the substrate, and if the substrate is more difficult to degrade, it might lead to a shift toward specific microbial groups that are more capable of handling that complexity, like the hydrolytic and acetogenic bacteria [19].

3.1.3 Temperature: Mesophilic vs. thermophilic

Under mesophilic conditions (30–40°C), the microbial community is more stable and diverse, typically favoring methanogenic bacteria. These conditions support a broad range of microbes, and the process tends to be more robust to fluctuations in substrate composition and operational conditions. Methanogens in the mesophilic range are generally more efficient at producing methane, making this the most common temperature range for anaerobic digestion processes.

When the temperature shifts to thermophilic conditions (50–60°C), microbial diversity typically decreases, and the overall microbial activity increases. Thermophilic bacteria, which can thrive at higher temperatures, are more efficient at breaking down organic matter quickly. However, higher temperatures can also make the process less stable due to the sensitivity of certain microbial groups to temperature fluctuations. In thermophilic conditions, the balance between hydrolytic, acetogenic, and methanogenic bacteria changes, and thermophilic methanogens become more dominant. This shift may increase the rate of methane production but can also lead to the rapid accumulation of VFAs if not carefully controlled [12, 20].

3.1.4 Carbon-to-nitrogen (C/N) ratio

The C/N ratio is a crucial factor in anaerobic digestion because it influences the nutrient balance available for microbial growth. A C/N ratio that is too high (excess carbon relative to nitrogen) can lead to a lack of nitrogen, which is essential for microbial protein synthesis. This limits microbial growth, especially for bacteria that participate in the later stages of digestion, including methane-producing methanogens. A balanced C/N ratio of around 20:1 to 30:1 is typically optimal for anaerobic digestion, as it ensures that microbes have enough nitrogen for growth without an overabundance of carbon, which can promote the production of excess VFAs. If the C/N ratio is too low, nitrogen becomes the limiting factor, potentially stunting microbial activity and reducing biogas production [13, 18, 21].

3.2 Impact of key environmental factors on methanogenic activity across diverse feedstocks: Experimental insights for optimizing biogas production

The efficiency of biogas production depends significantly on the activity of methanogens, which is influenced by various environmental factors. Methanogens are sensitive microorganisms, and their activity can fluctuate based on temperature, pH, nutrient availability, and the composition of the feedstock. To assess the impact of environmental variables like pH and salinity on methanogen activity across diverse feedstocks, a range of experimental approaches can be designed. These experiments would help determine how methanogenic archaea respond to changing environmental conditions in different substrates.

3.2.1 Temperature: The thermophilic vs. mesophilic

Temperature is a critical determinant of methanogenic activity. Methanogens typically thrive in two temperature ranges: mesophilic conditions (30–40°C) and thermophilic conditions (50–60°C). Experimental evidence suggests that thermophilic digestion leads to faster substrate breakdown and higher biogas yields due to enhanced microbial activity. However, thermophilic systems are more sensitive to fluctuations, requiring precise control to maintain stability. Mesophilic systems, on the other hand, are more robust and energy-efficient, making them suitable for a wider range of applications, especially in regions with limited resources for temperature regulation [8, 12, 16, 20, 22].

3.2.2 pH and alkalinity: Balancing the biochemical environment

The pH of the digestion environment plays a pivotal role in maintaining methanogenic activity. Methanogens perform optimally in a neutral to slightly alkaline pH range (6.8–7.5). Deviations from this range, either due to the accumulation of acids during acidogenesis or external factors, can inhibit methanogenic activity. Experimental interventions, such as the addition of alkaline buffers (e.g., calcium carbonate or sodium bicarbonate), have been shown to stabilize pH levels and enhance methane yields [16, 20].

3.2.3 Feedstock composition: Substrate diversity and nutrient balance

The composition of feedstock significantly influences methanogenic performance. Co-digestion of diverse substrates, such as food waste, agricultural residues, and wastewater sludge, provides an accelerating carbon-to-nitrogen (C:N) ratio, which is essential for optimal microbial activity. Experimental results indicate that a C:N ratio of 20–30:1 is ideal for maximizing biogas production. Additionally, the presence of inhibitors such as ammonia, sulfates, or heavy metals in certain feedstocks can suppress methanogenic activity. Pre-treatment methods, such as ammonia stripping or the use of microbial inhibitors, can mitigate these effects [22–24].

3.2.4 Trace nutrients and additives: Catalysts for enhanced methanogenesis

Methanogens require trace elements such as iron, cobalt, and nickel for enzyme function and metabolic pathways. Studies show that supplementation of these micronutrients in anaerobic digestion systems can significantly improve methane yields. For instance, the addition of iron has been found to stimulate the activity of hydrogenotrophic methanogens, leading to higher biogas output [16, 20, 22].

3.2.5 Hydraulic retention time (HRT) and organic loading rate (OLR)

The HRT and OLR are key operational parameters that influence methanogenic activity and biogas production. Experimental data indicate that an optimal balance between HRT and OLR ensures efficient substrate degradation without overloading the system. Prolonged HRT allows sufficient time for methanogens to process complex substrates, while an appropriate OLR prevents the accumulation of inhibitory by-products [16, 22, 23].

Visions from these experiments highlight the need for tailored approaches to anaerobic digestion, depending on the feedstock characteristics and environmental conditions. For instance:

- In regions with abundant agricultural residues, co-digestion with nutrient-rich substrates like food waste can address nutrient imbalances.

- For systems processing high-ammonia feedstocks, pre-treatment strategies, and microbial acclimation can enhance methanogenic tolerance.

Advanced monitoring tools can ensure real-time adjustments to pH, temperature, and loading rates, optimizing methanogenic activity.

By leveraging these experimental understandings, industry stakeholders can design and operate biogas systems that maximize efficiency, stability, and sustainability. The optimization of methanogenic activity across diverse feedstocks holds the key to unlocking the full potential of biogas as a renewable energy source [22, 23, 25].

4. Biogas: A sustainable energy solution powered by methanogens

4.1 Methanogens in sustainable energy

In the search for sustainable energy sources, biogas has emerged as a significant contender, due to the impressive efficiency of methanogens. These microorganisms are essential for anaerobic digestion, transforming organic waste into valuable energy through a complex and fascinating biochemical process.

Methanogens are a diverse group of archaea that thrive in oxygen-free environments, playing a critical role in the breakdown of organic matter. They can be found in various habitats, from wetlands to the digestive tracts of herbivores. These microorganisms have developed unique metabolic pathways that enable them to produce methane, the primary component of biogas. The importance of methanogens in renewable energy and biogas production cannot be overstated, as they facilitate the conversion of waste into energy and help reduce greenhouse gas emissions [3, 23, 25].

4.2 The process of biogas production

Biogas production consists of multiple stages, beginning with the breakdown of complex organic materials. The first phase is hydrolysis, where larger organic molecules are decomposed into simpler compounds through the action of enzymes. This is followed by acidogenesis, during which anaerobic bacteria convert these simpler compounds into organic acids, hydrogen, and carbon dioxide. The final stage, methanogenesis, is where methanogens shine. They use the by-products from earlier processes to produce methane and carbon dioxide. This biogas can be harvested for various applications, making it a versatile renewable energy source.

The combustion of biogas can produce electricity and heat, while upgraded biogas, known as biomethane, can be used as vehicle fuel, providing a cleaner alternative to fossil fuels [8, 23].

4.3 Applications of biogas

Biogas has multiple applications, including:

Electricity generation: Biogas can be used in gas engines or turbines to generate electricity. This is especially beneficial for rural areas or farms where organic waste is plentiful, providing a decentralized energy solution and reducing dependence on fossil fuels.

Heating: Biogas can be directly burned in boilers for heating, offering an efficient means to heat residential and commercial spaces, as well as for industrial processes.

Vehicle fuel: With appropriate upgrades, biogas can be transformed into biomethane, a clean-burning alternative to natural gas. This application holds promise in the transportation sector, where the demand for sustainable fuel options is increasing.

Fertilizer production: The leftover digestate from anaerobic digestion is nutrient-rich and can be used as organic fertilizer, returning valuable minerals to the soil, and promoting sustainable agricultural practices [23, 26, 27].

4.4 Environmental benefits, challenges, and comparative insights on biogas

4.4.1 Environmental benefits of biogas

Biogas production offers significant environmental advantages by utilizing methanogens to convert organic waste into energy. This process reduces the volume of waste sent to landfills, alleviating pressure on waste management systems and curbing the release of methane—a potent greenhouse gas generated during landfill decomposition. Moreover, biogas production supports the principles of a circular economy by transforming waste into valuable resources like energy and fertilizers. This reduces resource consumption and enhances sustainability [24, 28].

4.4.2 Challenges in biogas adoption

Despite its benefits, the widespread adoption of biogas faces several challenges. Technical issues, such as optimizing anaerobic digestion systems and managing diverse feedstocks, require innovative solutions. Additionally, public awareness about biogas' potential and the pivotal role of methanogens in sustainable energy systems need to be amplified. Addressing these challenges is essential to unlocking the full potential of biogas as a renewable energy source [28].

Future research is likely to focus on improving the efficiency of methanogens and developing innovative operational strategies for anaerobic digestion. Advances in synthetic biology and genetic engineering may open new avenues for optimizing microbial activity, potentially increasing biogas yields and enhancing overall system performance [28, 29].

4.5 Comparative insights on biogas and other renewable energy sources

Renewable energy is essential for mitigating climate change, enhancing energy security, and promoting sustainable development. Key sources such as biogas, ethanol, biodiesel, and solar energy each contribute uniquely while facing specific limitations.

DOI: http://dx.doi.org/10.5772/intechopen.1009384

This section compares biogas with other renewable energy sources based on energy content, feedstock requirements, greenhouse gas emissions, infrastructure needs, production costs, and environmental impacts. The analysis highlights the distinctive advantages of biogas, particularly its role in waste management and greenhouse gas mitigation [23–25, 30]. By harnessing the complementary strengths of various renewable energy technologies, a diversified and resilient energy portfolio can be established to sustainably meet future energy demands [26].

4.5.1 Energy content

Biogas has a lower energy content and density compared to ethanol and biodiesel. However, it remains a versatile energy source, suitable for heating, electricity generation, and as a vehicle fuel when purified or compressed. In contrast, solar energy does not produce fuel but generates electricity, which can either be stored in batteries or fed directly into power grids. The efficiency of each energy source varies depending on the application and specific end-user needs [23, 31].

4.5.2 Feedstock sustainability

Biogas relies on waste streams, making it a circular economy solution and preventing landfill methane emissions. It transforms waste streams into energy while addressing waste management challenges. Biochemically, the anaerobic digestion process involves the breakdown of organic matter by microorganisms, producing methane and carbon dioxide. This process is sensitive to pH, temperature, and feedstock composition, which influence its efficiency and scalability. Biogas systems are particularly advantageous in regions with abundant organic waste and limited agricultural land [26].

Ethanol is produced from corn and sugarcane, and ethanol's reliance on crops introduces concerns about food security and land competition. The biochemical fermentation process used in ethanol production requires significant water and energy inputs, leading to environmental trade-offs. Land-use changes for ethanol crops can lead to deforestation and biodiversity loss, further intensifying its environmental impact [26].

Biodiesel is derived from vegetable oils and animal fats, biodiesel production faces similar sustainability challenges as ethanol due to its dependence on agricultural resources, resource competition and the environmental costs of crop cultivation. The transesterification process used in biodiesel production requires chemical catalysts, which can generate hazardous waste. Furthermore, the reliance on monoculture crops contributes to soil degradation and reduces biodiversity.

Solar energy uses sunlight, an inexhaustible resource, but its reliance on mined materials for panel production raises concerns about resource depletion and the environmental impacts of mining activities. The scalability of solar energy systems is often constrained by the availability of rare earth metals and the need for sustainable recycling technologies.

4.5.3 Greenhouse gas emissions

Biogas has a low greenhouse gas (GHG) emission profile, particularly when methane is captured and utilized effectively, preventing its release into the atmosphere. This reduces its global warming potential significantly.

Conversely, ethanol and biodiesel emit CO_2 during combustion and have significant indirect emissions due to land-use changes, deforestation, and high fertilizer use, which can release nitrous oxide (a potent greenhouse gas). Solar energy, while emission-free during operation, involves lifecycle emissions associated with panel manufacturing, transportation, and disposal. Addressing these lifecycle emissions through green manufacturing practices and recycling programs is essential to minimize environmental trade-offs [20, 23, 26].

4.5.4 *Infrastructure requirements*

Biogas: Requires digesters and gas storage systems. These systems are scalable and suitable for decentralized energy production and well-suited for decentralized energy production in rural and urban settings. However, the initial investment and operational maintenance can be barriers to widespread adoption, particularly in developing regions. Technological advancements in bioreactor designs and feedstock preprocessing can improve scalability.

Ethanol: Relies on distilleries, which are capital-intensive and energy demanding, posing challenges for scalability. Additionally, the concentration of ethanol production in specific regions can strain local water resources and infrastructure.

Biodiesel: Requires refineries that demand substantial resources and infrastructure, often limiting their feasibility in resource-constrained regions. The environmental impact of these facilities can be mitigated through the adoption of cleaner production technologies and sustainable sourcing of feedstocks.

Solar energy: Involves solar panels, inverters, and sometimes battery storage. While simpler and increasingly cost-effective, large-scale solar installations may require significant land, raising potential land-use conflicts. Urban solar installations, such as rooftop panels, can alleviate some scalability challenges but may not meet large-scale energy demands.

4.5.5 *Production cost*

Biogas systems are moderately expensive to establish but offer long-term cost benefits, especially for facilities with abundant organic waste. Innovations in biogas purification and storage technologies can further reduce costs and enhance scalability. Ethanol and biodiesel production are costly due to their reliance on agricultural inputs and energy-intensive refining processes. Solar energy, though increasingly cost-competitive, often depends on government incentives or subsidies to offset initial installation expenses. The development of efficient recycling systems for solar panels could also reduce lifecycle costs and enhance environmental sustainability.

4.5.6 *Environmental impact*

Biogas effectively addresses waste management and pollution issues, offering a dual benefit of energy production and environmental conservation. Its role in reducing methane emissions and providing renewable energy makes it a critical component of climate change mitigation strategies. Ethanol and biodiesel, while renewable, are associated with unsustainable agricultural practices, including water-intensive crop cultivation and fertilizer overuse, which contribute to soil degradation and water scarcity. Biodiesel's land-use impacts, such as deforestation and habitat loss, further highlight its environmental trade-offs. Solar energy, with minimal operational impact, requires sustainable solutions for managing land-use and recycling panels at the end of their lifecycle. Advances in panel design, such as the use of less toxic materials and improved energy efficiency, could significantly reduce its environmental footprint.

4.6 Broader environmental implications

Biogas not only mitigates waste but also enhances soil health by providing nutrient-rich digestate as a byproduct, which can be used as organic fertilizer. This contributes to sustainable agriculture by reducing dependence on synthetic fertilizers. Ethanol and biodiesel production, while renewable, exacerbate water scarcity and can disrupt local ecosystems due to pesticide runoff and nutrient leaching into water bodies. The environmental implications of solar energy include habitat disruption from large installations and the challenges associated with end-of-life panel disposal. Developing circular economy solutions for panel recycling and utilizing brownfields for installations can mitigate these impacts [32].

5. Innovative technologies in biogas production

The field of biogas production has witnessed significant advancements in recent years, driven by the need to maximize yield, improve efficiency, and enhance sustainability. Several innovative technologies and methodologies have emerged, positioning biogas as a crucial player in renewable energy and waste management systems. New techniques like co-digestion, where multiple organic substrates are digested together, have been shown to increase biogas yields. Advanced biogas upgrading systems, such as membrane separation, allow for the purification of biogas to natural gas standards [8].

5.1 Co-digestion for enhanced biogas yields

Co-digestion is an emerging technique that involves the simultaneous digestion of multiple organic substrates, such as food waste, agricultural residues, and wastewater sludge, in the same anaerobic digestion system. Co-digestion of mixed substrates increases biogas yields by optimizing nutrient balance and microbial activity. Application in municipal waste management and agriculture demonstrates cost-effectiveness and efficiency [17, 28].

The advantages of co-digestion systems can be summarized as follows:

- Higher biogas yields: Combining substrates with complementary characteristics, such as carbon-to-nitrogen ratios, enhances microbial activity and biogas production.

- Improved waste management: Co-digestion enables the effective treatment of various waste streams in one system, reducing disposal challenges.

- Cost-effectiveness: By processing multiple wastes together, facilities can achieve economies of scale and reduce operational costs.

- Applications: Municipal waste treatment plants and agricultural biogas facilities increasingly employ co-digestion to improve efficiency and profitability [17, 28, 33].

5.2 Advanced biogas upgrading systems

Raw biogas contains impurities like carbon dioxide (CO_2), hydrogen sulfide (H_2S), and water vapor, which limit its direct use. Advanced upgrading technologies have been developed to purify biogas into biomethane, a renewable substitute for natural gas. Key methods include:

Membrane separation: A highly efficient technique that uses selective membranes to separate methane (CH_4) from other gases. Advantages include compact design, scalability, and low energy consumption [17, 28, 34].

Pressure swing adsorption (PSA): Removes CO_2 and other impurities by cycling gas through absorbent materials under varying pressure. PSA offers high purification efficiency and is widely adopted in large-scale facilities [17, 34].

Water scrubbing and chemical absorption: These technologies use water or chemical solutions to absorb impurities, yielding high purity biomethane [17, 34].

Cryogenic separation: Is an innovative technique that cools biogas to effectively separate its components at their condensation points. This method results in high-quality biomethane and facilitates the recovery of valuable by-products such as liquid CO_2 [17, 34].

6. Economic feasibility and lifecycle analysis of advanced biogas technologies

To validate the scalability and sustainability of advanced biogas technologies, a detailed assessment of their economic feasibility and lifecycle impact is essential:

Economic feasibility: Initial investment and operational costs vary significantly between upgrading methods. Membrane separation and PSA offer lower operational costs and higher energy efficiency, making them more suitable for mid to large-scale operations.

Cryogenic separation, although capital-intensive, provides opportunities for revenue generation through the sale of by-products like liquid CO_2. The ability to monetize these by-products can offset the higher initial costs and make the technology viable in the long-term.

Integration with renewable energy sources, such as solar or wind power, can further reduce operational costs by providing a sustainable energy supply for upgrading processes [26, 27, 35].

Life-cycle analysis (LCA): Comprehensive LCAs reveal that biogas upgrading technologies significantly reduce greenhouse gas emissions compared to fossil fuel usage. For instance, replacing natural gas with biomethane derived from upgraded biogas can cut carbon footprints by up to 90%.

Biogas systems contribute to waste reduction by diverting organic waste from landfills and reducing methane emissions from decomposition.

Circular economy principles are evident in these technologies, as they not only produce clean energy but also recover valuable resources like nutrients and carbon dioxide [26, 27, 34, 35].

Scalability and adaptability: Advanced biogas technologies can be adapted to different scales, from small agricultural setups to large municipal treatment facilities. Modular designs, particularly in membrane separation systems, allow for phased expansions as demand grows.

Policy incentives, such as carbon credits and subsidies for renewable energy production, enhance the economic feasibility of adopting these technologies globally [26, 27, 32, 34, 35].

By addressing both economic and environmental dimensions, advanced biogas production and upgrading technologies ensure not only enhanced energy yields but also long-term sustainability, making them a cornerstone of modern renewable energy solutions.

7. Challenges and future directions in biogas production

Despite advancements, biogas production faces significant challenges that require innovative solutions. Methanogens, the microorganisms central to biogas production, are highly sensitive to environmental factors such as temperature, pH, and substrate composition. These factors affect metabolic activity and the stability of anaerobic digestion systems. Additionally, the high initial capital and operational costs of constructing and maintaining digesters pose barriers to adoption, especially for small-scale operators.

To tackle these challenges effectively, it is important to examine the core issues impacting biogas systems and explore cutting-edge solutions. Addressing technical and biological challenges is key to overcoming these hurdles and ensuring sustainable advancements [29, 34].

7.1 Addressing technical and biological challenges

The sensitivity of methanogens and the complexities of AD systems necessitate advanced approaches to ensure stability and efficiency. These include:

Advanced biotechnological approaches: Genetic engineering of methanogens offers solutions to improve AD performance. Enhanced strains can withstand environmental stresses such as high-ammonia concentrations, maintaining stability and efficiency under diverse conditions. For instance, overexpression of key enzymes in the methanogenesis pathway, such as methyl-coenzyme M reductase, has shown promise in improving methane yield. Tools like CRISPR-Cas9 enable precise genome editing, fostering the development of robust methanogen strains [36].

Tailored microbial consortia: Synergistic microbial consortia, combining cellulolytic bacteria and methanogens, accelerating the breakdown of lignocellulosic biomass, addressing feedstock variability issues and enhancing biogas production efficiency [13, 29].

Process optimization: Co-digestion of multiple feedstock types and real-time monitoring of AD system parameters optimize efficiency and stability. Advanced monitoring systems with integrated sensor technologies and data analytics ensure rapid detection and correction of imbalances [8].

Smart monitoring and control systems: The use of sensors, Internet of Things (IoT) devices, and machine learning algorithms in anaerobic digestion systems has revolutionized biogas production:

- Real-time monitoring: Advanced sensors track key parameters such as pH, temperature, and gas composition, ensuring optimal reactor performance.

- Predictive maintenance: AI-based systems can predict equipment failures, reducing downtime and maintenance costs.

- Dynamic optimization: Machine learning algorithms optimize feedstock mixtures and process conditions to maximize biogas yields [37].

7.2 Emerging research trends: Expanding horizons in biogas technology

Emerging research trends are shaping the future of biogas production, with a focus on integrating biogas systems into broader environmental and energy strategies:

Methanogens in carbon capture and storage (CCS): Methanogens are gaining attention for their potential role in carbon capture and storage (CCS). These microorganisms can convert CO_2 into methane under anaerobic conditions, enabling simultaneous renewable energy production and greenhouse gas reduction. Research focuses on enhancing CO_2 conversion efficiency through genetic modifications and optimized reactor designs. Integrating biogas systems with CCS technologies could transform anaerobic digestion into a dual-purpose solution for mitigating climate change and providing sustainable energy [38].

Microbial electrochemical systems (MES): Innovations in MES enable the direct use of electricity to drive microbial methane production from CO_2 and hydrogen. This approach has potential for integrating renewable electricity sources, such as wind or solar, with biogas production [39].

Valorization of by-products: Beyond biomethane, researchers are exploring ways to extract value from by-products of anaerobic digestion, such as biochar, digestate, and volatile fatty acids (VFAs). These by-products can be repurposed as soil amendments, feed additives, or chemical precursors, enhancing the overall economic and environmental viability of biogas systems [40].

Synthetic biology applications: Synthetic biology enables the design of custom microbial consortia tailored to specific feedstocks and operating conditions. Engineered microbes can be programmed to perform complex metabolic functions, such as enhanced degradation of lignocellulosic biomass or precise regulation of methanogenesis pathways.

Integration with circular economy principles: The development of closed-loop systems that integrate biogas production with waste management, agriculture, and energy sectors is gaining traction. These systems optimize resource use, reduce waste, and create synergistic benefits across industries [34, 39].

8. Integration with renewable energy systems

Innovative integration of biogas systems with other renewable energy technologies, such as solar and wind, enhances energy efficiency and reliability:

Hybrid systems: Biogas plants equipped with solar panels or wind turbines can meet the energy demands of auxiliary equipment like pumps and compressors. This integration ensures a consistent energy supply, even during periods when biogas production alone may not meet peak energy demands. For example, hybrid systems in rural regions can provide off-grid energy solutions, reducing reliance on fossil fuels and promoting energy equity [24, 41].

Power-to-gas technology: This technology uses surplus electricity from renewable sources to produce hydrogen *via* electrolysis, which is then injected into biogas reactors to produce methane through a biological or chemical methanation process. Power-to-gas systems offer a dual benefit: enhancing the calorific value of biogas and providing a storage solution for excess renewable electricity. Successful pilot projects in countries like Germany have demonstrated the potential of this approach in stabilizing energy grids and maximizing the utility of renewable energy [24, 41].

Energy hubs: Integrating biogas plants into larger renewable energy hubs that combine solar, wind, and biomass technologies can create synergistic benefits. These hubs can optimize resource use, reduce waste, and ensure a balanced energy supply throughout the year. Such systems also foster economic resilience by diversifying income streams for energy producers [24, 41].

The integration of biogas systems with other renewables underscores the importance of holistic energy strategies. By leveraging the unique strengths of each technology, hybrid systems can overcome individual limitations, reduce dependency on fossil fuels, and accelerate the global transition to sustainable energy.

9. Regulatory and policy frameworks supporting the adoption of methanogen-based technologies

The successful adoption and scaling of methanogen-based technologies for biogas production depend significantly on supportive regulatory and policy frameworks. As the renewable energy landscape continues to evolve, industry stakeholders, including biogas producers, technology developers, and investors, need clear guidelines and incentives to foster innovation and implementation [42].

Government incentives and subsidies: To accelerate the adoption of biogas technologies, many governments offer financial incentives such as grants, subsidies, and tax credits. These incentives are particularly important for covering the high initial capital costs associated with the construction of biogas plants and the implementation of advanced technologies. For example, subsidies for the installation of anaerobic digesters or biogas upgrading systems like membrane separation can lower entry barriers for smaller operators, enabling them to invest in innovative solutions. Policymakers should continue to expand these incentives to support the development of methanogen-based biogas systems that focus on maximizing efficiency and sustainability [38, 42, 43].

Carbon credit and emission reduction programs: Methanogen-based biogas systems play a vital role in reducing greenhouse gas emissions by capturing methane that would otherwise be released into the atmosphere from landfills or wastewater treatment plants. Regulatory frameworks that support carbon credit markets, such as the Clean Development Mechanism (CDM) or the European Union Emission Trading Scheme (EU ETS), provide biogas producers with financial returns for reducing emissions. By facilitating the trade of carbon credits, governments can incentivize investments in biogas systems and reward companies that adopt methanogen-based technologies that contribute to carbon sequestration [43, 44].

Renewable energy standards and renewable gas mandates: Many countries have established renewable energy targets, often requiring a certain percentage of energy to come from renewable sources. These standards can include provisions for the inclusion of biogas in the energy mix. Renewable gas mandates or guarantees of origin (GOs) allow biogas producers to prove the renewable origin of their gas and access premium markets. Such regulatory frameworks provide a stable market for biomethane, ensuring that the industry remains economically viable and competitive.

Additionally, aligning biogas production with national or regional renewable energy targets helps secure long-term investment in methanogen-based technologies [42].

Research and development support: Given the complexity of biogas production systems, especially those utilizing methanogens in the production of biomethane, ongoing research, and development are essential for addressing technical challenges and advancing system efficiency. Governments and international organizations can foster R&D by funding academic and industrial research projects, providing grants for pilot programs, and facilitating collaboration between the public and private sectors. Policy frameworks that prioritize research into the genetic engineering of methanogens, optimization of anaerobic digestion processes, and integration of biogas with other renewable energy technologies will accelerate technological advancements [23, 29, 42].

Waste management and circular economy policies: Methanogen-based technologies have the dual benefit of providing renewable energy while addressing waste management challenges. By incentivizing the use of organic waste streams such as agricultural residues, food waste, and wastewater sludge, policymakers can align biogas production with circular economy principles. Waste diversion policies that promote the use of organic waste for biogas production, such as landfill diversion mandates or organic waste recycling laws, create an enabling environment for the adoption of methanogen-based biogas systems. These policies reduce waste and contribute to a cleaner, more sustainable environment while supporting the growth of the biogas industry [26, 32, 42].

Streamlined permitting and regulatory approvals: The permitting process for biogas projects can often be cumbersome and time-consuming, deterring potential investors. Simplified and expedited permitting procedures are essential to ensure that biogas projects can be implemented quickly and efficiently. Policymakers can help by creating clear, transparent, and standardized regulations for biogas projects, particularly for small-scale systems or pilot projects. This includes setting guidelines for site selection, environmental impact assessments, and safety protocols to ensure that biogas projects meet regulatory requirements without excessive delay [42].

Public-private partnerships (PPPs): Industry stakeholders can also benefit from public-private partnerships (PPPs) that facilitate the adoption of methanogen-based biogas technologies. These partnerships allow for the pooling of resources, expertise, and risk-sharing between governments and private enterprises. For instance, joint ventures can support large-scale biogas projects that incorporate the latest technological innovations and provide training, capacity building, and access to international markets. Governments can contribute to these partnerships by providing infrastructure support, regulatory guidance, and long-term policy stability [42, 45, 46].

9.1 Practical perspective for industry stakeholders

For industry stakeholders, navigating the regulatory landscape and leveraging these supportive frameworks is key to successful implementation. Investors and technology developers should stay informed about changes in policy incentives, carbon credit schemes, and renewable energy targets to align their strategies with emerging opportunities. Collaboration with policymakers can ensure that the necessary regulatory frameworks are in place to support the deployment of methanogen-based technologies at scale.

Furthermore, building partnerships with academic institutions and research organizations can help industry stakeholders stay at the forefront of technological innovations. By engaging in joint research initiatives or participating in pilot projects, companies can assess innovative solutions in real-world settings, refine their technologies, and build a competitive edge [46].

10. Case study: Analysis of methanogenic populations in OFMSW treatment

As mentioned earlier, methanogens play a crucial role in biogas production. These microorganisms break down organic matter into methane and carbon dioxide, providing a renewable energy source and addressing global waste management challenges. Among various applications, the anaerobic digestion (AD) of the organic fraction of municipal solid waste (OFMSW) is a biologically optimizable process with significant potential for sustainable energy production.

This part delves into the importance of methanogens in AD, focusing on a case study that highlights microbial population dynamics in two parallel digesters treating OFMSW. It explores the relationship between methanogen diversity, environmental conditions, and methane yield to demonstrate how bioindicators can enhance digestion performance.

10.1 Overview

A key industrial case study analyzed microbial balance in two pilot-scale anaerobic digesters operated by ACEA Pineries Industriale. ACEA is a modern multi-utility company that processes 60,000 tonnes per year of the organic fraction of municipal solid waste (OFMSW), serving approximately 1 million residents. The thermophilic digestion process, maintained at 55 ± 1 °C, occurs within two parallel biodigesters, referred to as Reactor A and Reactor B. Both digesters had identical designs and were fed the same OFMSW, except for the inclusion of a biopolymer additive in one system. The aim was to assess how the additive influenced methanogenic communities and methane yield [47]. The results revealed a decrease in total methanogen abundance and activity with the additive inclusion:

- Total methanogens decreased from 7.67 to 7.48 Log gene copies/mL sludge.

- Methanobactin spp., the most dominant methanogen, declined from 6.05 to 5.69 Log gene copies/mL sludge (T-test $p < 0.01$).

This reduction correlated with a slight decline in methane yield (−8%), indicating that while Methanobactin played a dominant role, the broader methanogenic community was highly heterogeneous and complex. The study underscored that variations in methanogen populations can act as bioindicators of digestion performance. Even slight modulations in key methanogens like Methanobactin can impact methane production. However, only a fraction of the active methanogens was characterized, highlighting the need for further research to fully understand the microbial interactions within digesters [47].

10.2 Implications and applications

The findings from this case study provide several key insights:

- Optimization potential: Understanding methanogen dynamics can improve digester performance by enabling targeted interventions, such as additive selection or feedstock adjustments.

- Sustainability: The use of OFMSW in AD offers a sustainable pathway for waste management and renewable energy production, reducing reliance on fossil fuels.

- Bioindicators: Methanogen population shifts serve as valuable bioindicators, offering a predictive tool for digestion efficiency under varying conditions.

This research demonstrates the critical role of methanogens in advancing sustainable anaerobic digestion technologies. Future work should focus on characterizing the full methanogenic community and further exploring genetic or biochemical interventions to enhance methane yields [47].

11. Conclusion

Methanogens are pivotal to the sustainable energy landscape, driving the production of biogas—a renewable energy source with vast potential. As the world seeks to transition toward more sustainable energy solutions, understanding and harnessing the power of these microorganisms will be key to unlocking a cleaner, greener future. With advancements in biogas technologies, including co-digestion, advanced upgrading systems, and integration with renewable energy sources, biogas is positioned to play a critical role in addressing global energy demands and waste management challenges [24, 29, 32].

The future of biogas lies in continued innovation. Technologies like smart monitoring and control systems are optimizing biogas production by enhancing efficiency and reducing operational costs. Advanced approaches in biotechnology, such as genetic engineering and tailored microbial consortia, are improving process stability, and increasing biogas yields. These innovations, combined with the adoption of circular economy principles, help ensure that biogas systems not only provide clean energy but also recover valuable resources, further advancing sustainability goals [37, 48].

To fully realize the potential of biogas, a unified vision for innovation and collaboration is essential. Addressing economic, technical, and regulatory challenges requires coordinated strategies that include increased funding for research, incentives for biogas adoption, and the establishment of supportive policy frameworks. Collaboration among researchers, industry stakeholders, and policymakers will be key to overcoming these barriers and scaling biogas systems for widespread use [29, 49].

Regulatory frameworks and policies play a critical role in enabling the adoption of methanogen-based biogas technologies. Government incentives, carbon credit markets, renewable energy standards, and research funding all contribute to creating an environment that supports biogas production. Policies that encourage waste diversion, streamline permitting processes, and incentivize public-private partnerships will further enhance the scalability and economic viability of biogas systems. By fostering such supportive frameworks, industry stakeholders can confidently invest in and implement innovative technologies, accelerating the transition to a sustainable energy future [29, 42, 43].

By leveraging innovative technologies and fostering a collaborative environment, biogas production can evolve into a scalable, reliable, and sustainable component of global renewable energy and waste management systems. This will not only contribute to energy independence but also promote environmental stewardship, ensuring a healthier planet for future generations [34].

In conclusion, methanogens and biogas production are central to the renewable energy transition. Through innovation, collaboration, and a commitment to sustainability, biogas can become a cornerstone of our global energy solutions—driving cleaner, greener, and more resilient communities.

Acknowledgements

The author acknowledges the use of ChatGPT for language editing in the chapter. I dedicate this chapter to the loving memory of my sister, Sormeh. I embarked on this journey during the incredibly tough time of her passing, yet her unwavering strength, compassion, and wisdom inspire me every day. Just as methanogens quietly transform waste into energy, creating new life from what seems depleted, Sormeh's spirit reminds me that resilience and hope can emerge even in the most challenging moments. This work is not only a reflection of scientific discovery but also a tribute to her lasting impact and presence in my life.

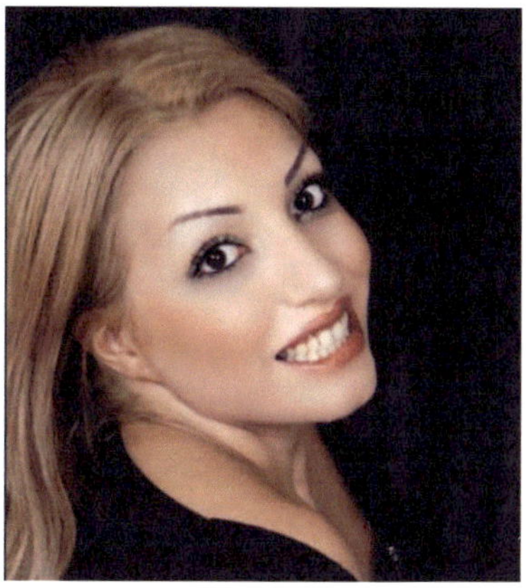

Sormeh Chegini (Feb 1985–Feb 2024).

Author details

Salomeh Chegini
Toronto Metropolitan University, George Brown College, Toronto, Canada

*Address all correspondence to: salomeh.chegini@torontomu.ca

References

[1] Marić A-K, Sudar M, Findrik Blažević Z, Vuković Domanovac M. Methanogenesis—General principles and application in wastewater remediation. Energies. 2024;**17**(21):5374

[2] Kharitonov S, Semenov M, Sabrekov A, Kotsyurbenko O, Zhelezova A, Schegolkova N. Microbial communities in methane cycle: Modern molecular methods gain insights into their global ecology. Environments. 2021;**8**(2):16

[3] Ray S, Kuppam C, Pandit S, Kumar P. Biogas upgrading by hydrogenotrophic methanogens: An overview. Waste and Biomass Valorization. 2023;**14**(2):537-552

[4] Harirchi S, Wainaina S, Sar T, Nojoumi SA, Parchami M, Parchami M, et al. Microbiological insights into anaerobic digestion for biogas, hydrogen or volatile fatty acids (VFAs): A review. Bioengineered. 2022;**13**(3):6521-6557

[5] Lyu Z, Shao N, Akinyemi T, Whitman WB. Methanogenesis. Current Biology. 2018;**28**(13):R727-RR32

[6] Ferry JG. Fundamentals of methanogenic pathways that are key to the biomethanation of complex biomass. Current Opinion in Biotechnology. 2011;**22**(3):351-357

[7] Whitman WB, Bowen TL, Boone DR. The methanogenic bacteria. Prokaryotes. 2006;**3**(Chapter 9):165-207

[8] Kelif Ibro M, Ramayya Ancha V, Beyene Lemma D. Biogas production optimization in the anaerobic Codigestion process: A critical review on process parameters modeling and simulation tools. Journal of Chemistry. 2024;**2024**(1):4599371

[9] Chegini S, Elbeshbishy E. Enhancing single-and two-stage anaerobic digestion of thickened waste-activated sludge through FNA-heat pretreatment. Processes. 2024;**12**(2):345

[10] Pasalari H, Gholami M, Rezaee A, Esrafili A, Farzadkia M. Perspectives on microbial community in anaerobic digestion with emphasis on environmental parameters: A systematic review. Chemosphere. 2021;**270**:128618

[11] Su X, Li D, Xia D, Zhao W, Fu H, Guo H. Laboratory study on microbial fractionation mechanisms of carbon and hydrogen isotopes in coalbed biomethane. AAPG Bulletin. 2023;**107**(9):1493-1515

[12] Maddela NR, Aransiola SA, Ezugwu CI, Eller LKW, Scalvenzi L, Meng F. Microbial Biotechnology for Bioenergy. Elsevier; 2024

[13] Tyagi VK, Bhatia A, Kubota K, Rajpal A, Ahmed B, Khan AA, et al. Microbial community dynamics in anaerobic digesters treating organic fraction of municipal solid waste. Environmental Technology and Innovation. 2021;**21**:101303

[14] Liu J, Tang Z, Wang C, Wu K, Song Y, Wang X, et al. Novel technique for sustainable utilisation of water hyacinth using EGSB and MCSTR: Control overgrowth, energy recovery, and microbial metabolic mechanism. Renewable Energy. 2021;**163**:1701-1710

[15] Singh N, Singh V, Singh MP. Microbial degradation of lignocellulosic biomass for bioenergy production: A metagenomic-based approach. Biocatalysis and Biotransformation. 2023;**41**(1):15-25

[16] Shukla S, Rai S, Senthamizh R, Sahoo S, Yadav P, Mal J. Municipal solid waste management and effect of process parameters on the treatment methods. In: Solid Waste Management. 1st edition. CRC Press; 2024. p. 20. eBook ISBN: 9781003229919

[17] Saboohi Z, Hosseini SE. Advancements in biogas production: Process optimization and innovative plant operations. Clean Energy. © 2025 National Institute of Clean-and-Low-Carbon Energy. 2025:zkae096. Online ISSN 2515-396X. Print ISSN 2515-4230

[18] Mao C, Wang Y, Wang X, Ren G, Yuan L, Feng Y. Correlations between microbial community and C:N:P stoichiometry during the anaerobic digestion process. Energy. 2019;**174**:687-695

[19] Kamperidou V, Terzopoulou P. Anaerobic digestion of lignocellulosic waste materials. Sustainability. 2021;**13**(22):12810

[20] Induchoodan T, Haq I, Kalamdhad AS. Factors affecting anaerobic digestion for biogas production: A review. In: Advanced Organic Waste Management. Elsevier; 2022. pp. 223-233

[21] Laiq Ur Rehman M, Iqbal A, Chang CC, Li W, Ju M. Anaerobic digestion. Water Environment Research. 2019;**91**(10):1253-1271

[22] Ajayi-Banji A, Rahman S. A review of process parameters influence in solid-state anaerobic digestion: Focus on performance stability thresholds. Renewable and Sustainable Energy Reviews. 2022;**167**:112756

[23] Czekała W. Biogas as a Sustainable and Renewable Energy Source. In: Di Blasio G, Agarwal AK, Belgiorno G, Shukla PC, editors. Clean Fuels for Mobility. Energy, Environment, and Sustainability. Singapore: Springer; 2022. DOI: 10.1007/978-981-16-8747-1_10

[24] Calise F, Cappiello FL, Cimmino L, d'Accadia MD, Vicidomini M. A review of the state of the art of biomethane production: Recent advancements and integration of renewable energies. Energies. 2021;**14**(16):4895

[25] Tariq MJA, Javed J, Habiba U, Meer S. Pioneering methanogens: the architects of modern eco-friendly renewable energy solutions [Internet]. Methanogens - Unique Prokaryotes [Working Title]. IntechOpen; 2025. DOI: 10.5772/intechopen.1008419

[26] Kabeyi MJB, Olanrewaju OA. Biogas production and applications in the sustainable energy transition. Journal of Energy. 2022;**2022**(1):8750221

[27] Ardolino F, Cardamone G, Parrillo F, Arena U. Biogas-to-biomethane upgrading: A comparative review and assessment in a life cycle perspective. Renewable and Sustainable Energy Reviews. 2021;**139**:110588

[28] Tagne RFT, Dong X, Anagho SG, Kaiser S, Ulgiati S. Technologies, challenges and perspectives of biogas production within an agricultural context. The case of China and Africa. Environment, Development and Sustainability. 2021;**23**:14799-14826

[29] Golmakani A, Nabavi SA, Wadi B, Manovic V. Advances, challenges, and perspectives of biogas cleaning, upgrading, and utilisation. Fuel. 2022;**317**:123085

[30] Kaitale F. Optimization of the Feedstocks for Biogas Process. 2024. Available from: https://urn.fi/URN:NBN:fi:aalto-202501221617

[31] Bakkaloglu S, Hawkes A. A comparative study of biogas and biomethane with natural gas and hydrogen alternatives. Energy and Environmental Science. 2024;**17**(4):1482-1496

[32] Chen R, Weng GM. Sustainable energy resources for driving methane conversion. Advanced Energy Materials. 2023;**13**(36):2301734

[33] Baena-Moreno FM, Sebastia-Saez D, Wang Q, Reina TR. Is the production of biofuels and bio-chemicals always profitable? Co-production of biomethane and urea from biogas as case study. Energy Conversion and Management. 2020;**220**:113058

[34] Sher F, Smječanin N, Hrnjić H, Karadža A, Omanović R, Šehović E, et al. Emerging technologies for biogas production: A critical review on recent progress, challenges and perspectives. Process Safety and Environmental Protection. 2024;**188**:834-859. DOI: 10.1016/j.psep.2024.05.138. Available from: https://www.sciencedirect.com/science/article/pii/S0957582024006608. ISSN 0957-5820

[35] Bruno M, Marchi M, Ermini N, Niccolucci V, Pulselli FM. Life cycle assessment and cost–benefit analysis as combined economic–environmental assessment tools: Application to an anaerobic digestion plant. Energies. 2023;**16**(9):3686

[36] Hemalatha P, Abda EM, Shah S, Prabhu SV, Jayakumar M, Karmegam N, et al. Multi-faceted CRISPR-Cas9 strategy to reduce plant based food loss and waste for sustainable bio-economy—A review. Journal of Environmental Management. 2023;**332**:117382

[37] Swami S, Suthar S, Singh R. et al. Integration of anaerobic digestion with artificial intelligence to optimise biogas plant operation. Environment, Development and Sustainability. 2023. DOI: 10.1007/s10668-023-04326-2

[38] Ravichandran M, Kumar TTA, Dineshkumar R. Carbon dioxide capture, sequestration, and utilization models for carbon management and transformation. Environmental Science and Pollution Research. 2024;**31**(44):55895-55916

[39] Das A, Dutta S. Sewage treatment & recovery of energy based on the integrated strategy of microbial electrochemical systems (MES). In: Shah MP, editors. Microbial Remediation of Hazardous Chemicals from Water & Industrial Wastewater Treatment Plant. Environmental Science and Engineering. Cham: Springer; 2024. DOI: 10.1007/978-3-031-62898-6_1

[40] Ribeiro AR, Devens KU, Camargo FP, Sakamoto IK, Varesche MBA, Silva EL. Synergizing sugarcane waste valorization: Optimization of two-stage anaerobic co-digestion for enhanced methane recovery and organic matter removal. Industrial Crops and Products. 2024;**221**:119297

[41] Mansouri SA, Nematbakhsh E, Ahmarinejad A, Jordehi AR, Javadi MS, Matin SAA. A multi-objective dynamic framework for design of energy hub by considering energy storage system, power-to-gas technology and integrated demand response program. Journal of Energy Storage. 2022;**50**:104206

[42] Agupugo CP, Ajayi AO, Nwanevu C, Oladipo SS. Policy and regulatory framework supporting renewable energy microgrids and energy storage systems. Engineering Science & Technology Journal. 2022;**5**:2589-2615

[43] Wara M, Victor DG. A realistic policy on international carbon offsets. Program

on Energy and Sustainable Development Working Paper. 2008;**74**:1-24

[44] Sutter C, Parreño JC. Does the current clean development mechanism (CDM) deliver its sustainable development claim? An analysis of officially registered CDM projects. Climatic Change. 2007;**84**(1):75-90

[45] Fleta-Asín J, Muñoz F. Renewable energy public–private partnerships in developing countries: Determinants of private investment. Sustainable Development. 2021;**29**(4):653-670

[46] Tapaninaho R, Heikkinen A. Value creation in circular economy business for sustainability: A stakeholder relationship perspective. Business Strategy and the Environment. 2022;**31**(6):2728-2740

[47] Negro V, Mainero D, Caredda C, Anedda E, Franchitti E, Traversi D. Analyses of methanogenic population as key Indicator for anaerobic digestion: A case-study in the organic fraction of municipal solid waste treatment. Waste and Biomass Valorization. 2023;**14**(8):2461-2468

[48] Bradu P, Biswas A, Nair C, Sreevalsakumar S, Patil M, Kannampuzha S, et al. Retracted Article: Recent advances in green technology and Industrial Revolution 4.0 for a sustainable future. Environmental Science and Pollution Research. Dec 2023;**30**(60):124488-519

[49] Eskandar K. Revolutionizing biotechnology and bioengineering: Unleashing the power of innovation. Journal Of Applied Biology & Biotechnology. 2023;**10**(3):81-88

Chapter 2

Pioneering Methanogens: The Architects of Modern Eco-Friendly Renewable Energy Solutions

Muhammad Junaid Ahmad Tariq, Jasia Javed, Ume Habiba and Sameen Meer

Abstract

Methanogens present a class of Archaea which are crucial for the production of biogas. The process involved in this type of energy production is the anaerobic digestion process which is a key component in contributing to the conversion of waste materials to useful energy materials, and it contributes to environmentally friendly renewable energy solutions. This chapter discusses the biological aspect, metabolic reactions, and pathways involved in converting organic waste into methane with the help of methanogens. Additionally, the role of methanogens as contributors toward sustainable alternative energy solutions and upgradation by various biotechnological, genetic engineering, and co-digestion approaches will be discussed. This helps to reduce the emission of greenhouse gases and to solve the problems related to climate and environmental changes. This chapter will also discuss the environmental impact of methanogen-based approaches for biogas production, utilization of waste resources, and waste treatment to contribute to green energy production. The contribution toward the growing importance and significance of renewable energy solutions will also be discussed, addressing technical challenges and possibly discussing the future potential of these organisms.

Keywords: methanogens, anaerobic digestion, biogas production, renewable energy, climate change mitigation, co-digestion, genetic engineering

1. Introduction

Methanogens are a particular group of microbes that are associated with the domain of Archaea. This group of microorganisms is particularly studied and well known for their ability to produce methane, which is an important bio-based fuel. The driving mechanism behind this methane production is a metabolic process known as methanogenesis. Methanogenesis occurs in an anaerobic, oxygen-free environment and can potentially occur in a variety of habitats, which can include landfills, working lands, and even the digestive tract of ruminant animals such as dairy animals (cows and goats) [1]. This process is carried out by methanogens, and the process plays a vital role in the carbon cycle by conversion of organic matter within waste materials into methane. This leads to the production of biogas, which is a renewable and sustainable energy alternative from biological resources [2].

The recent energy crisis has led to the discovery and consideration of various alternative energy resources. Methanogens have emerged as a possible alternative to traditional fossil fuel energy resources. The traditional fossil fuel energy resources are not only impacting the environment by climate changes, but there is a significant decrease in the global reserves of these nonrenewable energy resources, and this has disturbed the economic balance of various countries and has forced the policymakers to focus on sustainable energy alternatives that can address the issues of both environmental impact and depleting energy resources [3]. Hence in this regard, methanogens offer a unique solution to the underlying problem by utilizing organic base material for the production of clean alternative renewable energy resources, biogas. Additionally, the burning of biogas produces fewer greenhouse gases than conventional burning up close to the field such as coal and natural gas [4]. Another advantage of using biological production of renewable energy resources is the economic benefit that comes with the utilization of waste in producing biogas as an energy alternative. The impact of biological resources can be determined as a choice by various economic experts and policymakers as a possible alternative, as it balances economic instability by reducing the costs of waste treatment and increasing the production of energy simultaneously [5].

1.1 Methanogens: The natural sources of methane

As methanogens are a group of Archaea, they have distinct features from bacteria and hence involve several metabolic pathways, which allow them to thrive in diverse environmental conditions and be able to withstand high temperatures and extreme conditions. Hence, the methanogens can produce methane under three different temperature conditions that include lower temperature, optimized temperature, and high temperature [6]. In the range of optimized temperature, the best production of methane occurs, and this temperature is in the range of 30–40°C. However, as discussed earlier, the potential of methanogens to produce methane at different temperatures. They have the ability to produce methane and withstand diverse environmental conditions; due to the presence of these properties, they are widely used for biogas production [7]. Another characteristic feature of methanogens is their ability to provide methane in the absence of oxygen. Most organisms use oxygen for their respiratory purposes; however, methanogens are involved in anaerobic environments. Additionally, they can produce methane as a byproduct in the absence of oxygen. The ability of methanogens to convert carbon compounds results in the formation of byproduct methane. These carbon compounds included carbon dioxide and acetate. This process is a key parameter that is considered in the production of methane under various industrial processes. A series of complex biological processes and biochemical reactions contribute toward the production of methane by methanogenesis in this regard. The carbon dioxide and hydrogen molecules are utilized by methanogens and broken down through a series of processes to form methane and water as byproducts [8]. Moreover, methanogens can metabolize methyl amine compounds, acetates, and methanol eventually leading to the production of methane.

1.2 Methanogens in biogas production

There are four main steps involved in the production of methane by the process of methanogenesis. These four steps are points of consideration many researchers and

DOI: http://dx.doi.org/10.5772/intechopen.1008419

experts have often targeted these steps in order to maximize the production of biogas from methane. These four steps include hydrolysis, acidogenesis, acetogenesis, and finally methanogenesis, which is the step that yields methane [9]. Methane produced at the end of these steps is harnessed and used as a clean resource of energy for various purposes.

The process of anaerobic digestion can be carried out by various industrial processes such as wastewater treatment and agriculture waste management, all of these processes can contribute toward the production of biogas from organic waste materials. By utilization of the methanogenesis process in the waste treatment plants, the substrates and organic waste materials in the sludge are converted into biogas, which is then processed in such a way that they can then be used as a resource for the generation of electricity and headed for the industrial facility [10]. Likewise, agricultural-rich materials commonly manure, crop residues, and waste material from various vegetables and food wastes are processed, there will be conditions to produce biogas which is then utilized as an energy resource in rural areas.

The advantages of biogas over conventional fossil fuel energy resources are diverse. These renewable energy alternatives can not only be used for local production of energy, but they can also reduce the carbon footprint on a global scale [11]. The utilization of methane as a heat source from biogas produces a lesser amount of carbon dioxide compared to the amount released by burning fossil fuels. Additionally, the methane produced is captured and harnessed for the production of green energy, and hence its release into the environment is controlled, as it would otherwise act as a toxic greenhouse gas that has a considerably higher greenhouse effect compared to carbon dioxide [12].

1.3 Global significance and ecological effects

The increasing demand for energy sources, levels of population, and waste materials is a point to consider, as it is related to the changes in the environment and increased pollution rates. The utilization of sustainable energy alternatives is, however, an alternative approach to address all these issues and to produce a renewable form of energy that can be utilized in a renewable way [13]. This unique property of biological organisms is the reason why they are considered as eco-friendly alternatives to fossil fuels and waste management.

Anaerobic digestion is a highly beneficial process, not only for capturing methane as an energy source and preventing its release as a potent greenhouse gas but also for producing valuable byproducts. The materials generated after digestion are rich in natural nutrients that can be used as fertilizers, promoting plant growth and supporting sustainable agriculture [14]. These fertilizers offer cost-effective and better alternative to synthetic fertilizers.

The adaptability of biogas production via methanogenesis has a wide range of applications included, but are not restricted to the generation of electricity, production of heat, and as a transportation fuel in the form of compressed biomethane. This highlights the significance of biofuels as economic players and driving factors for the economic stability of a country [15]. As these renewable alternatives are cost-effective, they can be implemented at smaller scales as well as larger scales ranging from conventional household registers in small communities to large-scale industrial facilities making methanogenesis an easy cost-effective, and accessible energy option for diverse populations [16].

1.4 Current developments and technological innovations

There is a lot of potential for renewable energy resources toward addressing the issues that are faced in economical and environmental sectors. Despite this potential, various associated challenges need to be considered and optimized for the better performance of these renewable energy systems and not used as solutions for economic and environmental stability [17]. These issues can be addressed by recent advancements in the fields of biotechnology, genetic engineering, and biochemical processing. All these fields are focused on maximizing the amount of methane that is produced in the process of methanogenesis while ensuring the least production of other harmful substances that can potentially damage the environment. Additionally, these research approaches also focus on maximizing methane production by increasing the tolerance of microbes involved in diverse environments and extreme conditions [18]. One easy and cost-effective approach in this regard is the development of a co-digestion process where multiple substrates are processed by microbes, and this results in the production of methane. The advantage of this system is that it not only provides a diversity of multiple substrates but also the diversity of conditions for various microbial communities present in an anaerobic system so that they can work on the production of methane from waste [19]. This approach is being considered along with modifications, and it will be digestion conditions, bioreactor design, and retention capturing techniques for optimizing the overall methane production from resources.

2. Methanogens biology and ecology

As previously discussed, methanogens possess unique characteristics that make them an ideal candidate for the production of methane, a renewable energy source. In addition to this property, they also possess a variety of biological and ecological characteristics that help them to survive in extreme conditions. The production of biogas from methanogens is also accompanied by the production of anaerobic digester waste, which is an excellent resource of fertilizer for plants and can be processed to provide natural product-based products in replacement of conventional chemical fertilizers.

2.1 Classification of methanogens

Although methanogens fall under the domain Archaea, which is different from Bacteria and Eukarya, their characteristic features are main points to classify them further into several orders and families based on their phylogenetic relationships, metabolic pathways, and substrates used for methane production [20].

The main classes of methanogens include:

Methanobacteriales: In this order, Methanobacterium and Methanobrevibacter are some commonly understood methanogens [21]. The members of this group have the ability to utilize carbon dioxide as well as hydrogen for the production of methane and are typically named as hydrogenotrophic methanogens.

Methanococcales: This category of methanogens is also hydrogenotrophic, able to survive in complex environments and extreme conditions such as hot springs [22]. This group of methanogens is named Methanococcus methanogens.

Methanomicrobiales: The group of methanogens includes acetate-utilizing methanogens as well as hydrogenotrophic methanogens [23], as a result, they are both acetoclastic and hydrogenotrophic.

Methanopyrales: These are important species in geothermal ecosystems because they are high-temperature loving and are able to survive and produce methane in high-temperature conditions [24]. This class of methanogens is also useful in high heat-producing industrial processes.

Methanocalculus: The organisms of this order can grow and produce methane in environments of high salinity (**Figure 1**).

This classification of methanogens highlights the diversity of their work environments and their spread across various ecological systems. The adaptability of methanogens in varying conditions is the reason why they should be considered as a good alternative resource for the production of renewable energy [25].

2.2 Methanogenesis pathways

The pathways of methanogenesis involve the breakdown of various organic compounds into simpler compounds, and then these simpler compounds are further processed by various metabolic pathways, which lead to the production of methane [26] through the following key metabolic reactions:

Hydrogenotrophic methanogenesis: This is a methanogenesis process where the utilization of hydrogen and carbon dioxide results in the production of methane [27]. The organic waste that is used as a substrate for these types of reactions is first broken down into hydrogen and carbon dioxide, which are then converted into methane under with following Eq. (1).

$$4H2 + CO2 \rightarrow CH4 + 2H2O \quad (1)$$

This pathway commonly occurs in anaerobic environments where hydrogen is produced as a byproduct during the degradation of organic matter.

Acetoclastic methanogenesis: Under the conditions where acetate ions are produced [28], the methanogens adapt to acetoclastic methanogenesis. The overall reaction can be summarized using Eq. (2) as follows.

$$CH3COO- + H2O \rightarrow CH4 + CO2 \quad (2)$$

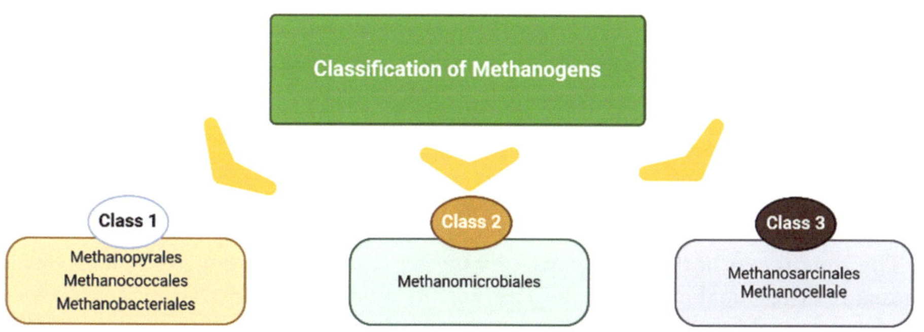

Figure 1.
Classification of methanogens.

Methylotrophic methanogenesis: In this type of reaction, methanol is primarily used as a substrate for the production of methane [29]. The methylated substrates produce methane through the following conversion reaction Eq. (3).

$$CH3OH \rightarrow CH4 + H2O \tag{3}$$

These types of reactions typically occur in marine sediments and during the degradation of organic matter.

The abovementioned pathways highlight the significant biochemical activity that is involved in the production of methane from its methanogenic classes. Over the years, the varying conditions and creating substrate types have pushed the methanogens toward genetic evolution, and hence these evolutions have resulted in the adaptability of methanogens over varying conditions for the production of methane.

2.3 Environmental niches and adaptation

The adaptability of methanogens in various environmental conditions stems from their ability to adapt to various stressful environments and changes in their genetic makeup through the process of evolution. These methanogens can work in various anaerobic conditions and in varying oxygen conditions, which marks their ecological success and diversity [30]. The diverse habitats of methanogens include:

Wetlands: The wetlands are composed of organic material and hence provide an ideal environment for the methanogens. These saturated soils are the ground for the decomposition of matter from animal and plant wastes and lead to significant methane production.

Landfills: The landfills are sites where the anaerobic conditions build up over time by accumulation of organic wastes, and this provides an environment for methanogens to work efficiently and produce methane. The methane produced in these processes is captured and used as biogas for the generation of energy.

Digestive tracts of ruminants: This is a natural phenomenon and occurs in the gastrointestinal tract of various ruminant animals. This has significance in terms of the digestive system of animals, as it helps to break down complex carbohydrates and is the fermentative process where methane is produced as a byproduct.

Hydrothermal vents: In the presence of high temperatures as well as high-pressure marine conditions such as those present in hydrothermal vents, methanogens are able to grow and produce methane through biogeochemical cycles.

Extreme salinity environments: Methanogens are able to survive in hypersaline conditions, which has marked their adaptability and allowed them to cover various ecological grounds which are otherwise uninhabitable by other microbial species (**Figure 2**).

2.4 Role of methanogens in the carbon cycle

The key process of methanogenesis by methanogens is a vital factor in addressing the issue of the global carbon cycle. The conversion of organic carbon to methane, which is released into the atmosphere or captured as biogas, has a significant impact in terms of environmental sustainability and the production of energy.

In natural ecosystems and controlled environments, methanogens can contribute to the utilization of organic waste matter to transform it into useful methane

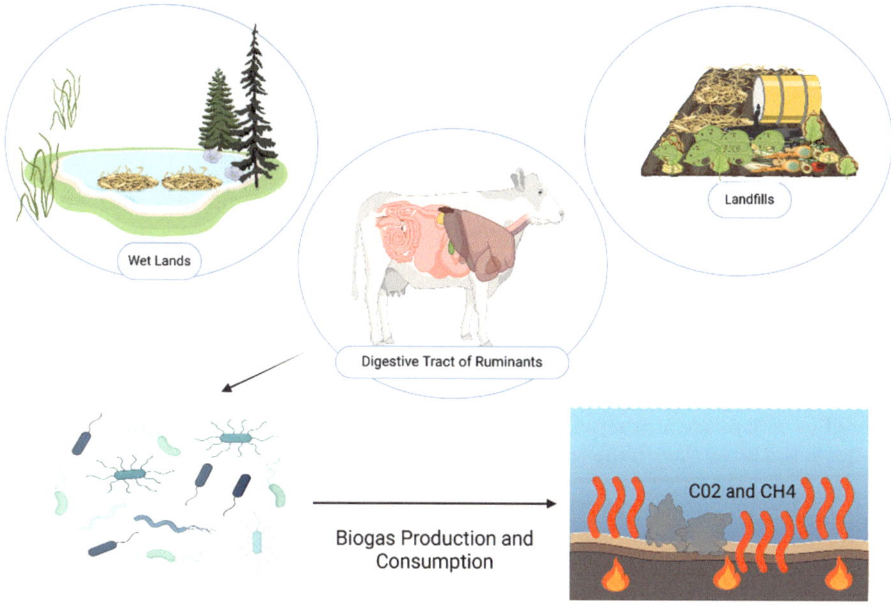

Figure 2.
Diversity of habitats for methanogens to thrive.

products. The carbon cycle in the natural ecosystem is also completed when methanol drops convert methane back into carbon dioxide. This leads to the completion of the carbon cycle, and an interplay between methanogens and methanotrophs is a key balance to maintain sustained levels of carbon in the environment [31]. Moreover, methane is more potent compared to carbon dioxide; it has a significantly less lifespan than carbon dioxide and hence contributes less toward climate change [32]. The capture and utilization of methane by various biogas systems are eventually helping the environment and reducing the production and emission of methane in the ecosystem.

3. Methanogens in renewable energy applications

The unique processes occurring in anaerobic systems have made methanogens an important class of microbes, highlighting their role in the production of energy through products produced during the anaerobic digestion process. The outline of the process is the introduction of microbes and waste materials in a specialized environment known as bioreactors in which controlled conditions are maintained. These components then undergo an anaerobic digestion process that over time converts the waste materials to byproducts and the methane is released through this process which is then collected, processed, and then stored in the form of biogas [33]. This section highlights the important role of methanogens in the production of biogas and their role in the generation of energy.

3.1 Biogas production

The anaerobic digestion process is one of the most important processes as it yields methane and involves the processing of organic waste matter from food waste, agricultural waste, and manure waste. Another important parameter in this process is the absence of oxygen, which enhances the metabolic activities of methanogens [34]. However, the process is broken down into a series of steps that occur consecutively throughout the whole process making sure that all the material is properly utilized in the process and that waste material is converted into useful byproducts.

Hydrolysis: The process of anaerobic digestion is continuous, and all the processes occur simultaneously meaning that at any particular time in a reactor, the process is undergoing different steps. However, the first stage of the process is the hydrolysis process, where the complex organic matter is broken down into simpler forms/compounds [35]. They are easily consumable products for the microbes that process these byproducts in the preceding stages of anaerobic digestion. The microbes involved in this process are hydrolytic bacteria and the enzymes that are involved in this process are hydrolytic enzymes are produced and released by these hydrolytic bacteria [36]. This is important because the process converts the complex carbohydrates, fats, and proteins present in the waste material into simpler sugars, fatty acids, and amino acids, which are easily soluble and act as byproducts for the next process.

Acidogenesis: The next process is acidogenesis, which utilizes the products of hydrolysis and further processes them to even shorter forms, comprising smaller chains of fatty acids, hydrogen molecules, CO_2, and alcohols via fermentation [37]. The bacteria involved in this process are acidogenic bacteria, and this is a crucial step the acidogenesis process yields the byproducts [38] which are then further consumed in the later part of the fermentative process. The acetogenesis acts as a platform for the methanogen bacteria for the production of methane.

Acetogenesis: This is the mixture of the elements from the fermentation process, where the acetogenic bacteria convert these short-chain fatty acids and alcohol-based products into acetate ions, hydrogen, and carbon dioxide. This process is fundamental, as it provides a setting stage for the methanogens [39], which consume these acetates as an imported substrate for the production of methane. Furthermore, the products of this process are also vital, as acetoclastic methanogenesis converts the acetates as substrates for the production of methane.

Methanogenesis: The final stage is ultimately the production of methane from the whole anaerobic digestion process and the key players in this process are methanogens, which convert the products of acetogenesis and acidogenesis (collectively called fermentation) into methane [40]. One particular point of consideration here is the utilization of substrates for the production of methane. Depending upon the availability of resources, the methanogens either use hydrogenotrophic, acetoclastic, or methylotrophic pathways, and this leads to variation in the amount of methane that is produced in the reaction (**Figure 3**).

The variation of production of methane in an anaerobic digestion process varies, and this depends upon various factors that include changes in pH, temperature, processing time, and the composition of waste material or organic feedstock that was used [41]. The process of anaerobic digestion yields biogas which is comprised of methane, carbon dioxide, and small amounts of other gases. The amount of methane is primarily 50–75% and the concentration of carbon dioxide is 25–50% while there is a 1% concentration of other gases [42]. The produced methane can then be purified through processing and can be used for electricity generation and heating or can we upgrade it to be used as vehicle fuel.

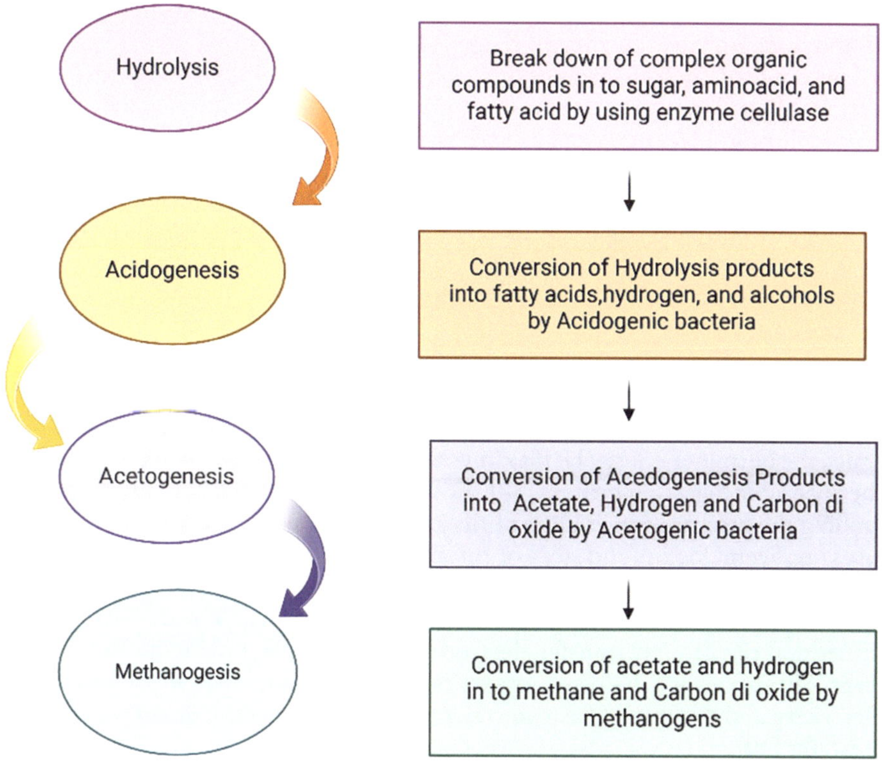

Figure 3.
Anaerobic digestion and methane production by methanogens.

3.2 Bioenergy generation

The generation of energy from biological systems represents an innovation in the field of energy production and an alternative to traditional methods. The product of methanogenesis yields methane [43], which can be processed for various purposes:

Electricity generation: One of the important purposes of biogas produced from methanogenesis is that it can be burned in systems known as combined heat and power (CHP) systems for the production of electricity [44]. These are high-efficiency systems that can convert approximately 90% of energy content from biogas into usable energy in the form of electricity. This is a useful approach as it minimizes the organic risk, maximizes its consumption, and maximizes the amount of energy that is produced through this organic waste.

Production of biofuel: Biofuel production is the process of upgrading biogas to produce biomethane. The main purpose of this process is to increase the methane content within the gas that is purified, allowing it to be used as a transportation fuel for combustion engines [45]. It is an increasing trend of modification and upgradation of biofuel production methods, maximizing the amount of methane so a bad trial mechanism can be used as a suitable alternative compared to fossil fuels, which have comparatively higher greenhouse gas emissions.

Grid injection: Another co-beneficial process involves the tradition of biogas to meet natural gas quality standards. This is helpful as produced biogas can then be injected into natural gas grids [46]. This practice can reduce the consumption of fossil fuels and increase the utilization of renewable energy resources.

Chemical feedstock: In terms of the useful products, yielded through anaerobic digestion, biogas is used as a combustible product while other intermediate products produced during this process can be used as feedstocks for the synthesis of various chemicals including hydrogen and other organic compounds [47]. This is an important point of process as it not only produces methane but also facilitates in production of various chemical products which holds significance in the bio-based economy.

3.3 Cutting-edge technologies using methanogens

The recent research focuses on the enhancement of the digestion process, as marked by the significance of the utilization of analytic techniques to enhance the useful properties of methanogens. The main purpose of these technologies is to enhance the output of energy by maximizing the production of methane at the end of the anaerobic digestion process [48]. However, this approach not only focuses on upgrading the methanogenesis step of the anaerobic digestion process, but it also focuses on several factors and steps of the anaerobic digestion process to achieve maximum methane at the end of the process.

Microbial fuel cells (MFCs): These fuel cells are composed of microbial communities that can directly transfer electrons to an electrode, producing an electric current. These fuel cells are being researched to be implemented for the production of electricity and to convert waste into electricity during the treatment process of wastewater [49].

Integrated anaerobic digestion systems: The main focus of these systems is to convert this material by combining waste management and treatment technologies with anaerobic digestion systems [50]. The utilization of these systems aims to enhance the interactions between different microbial species, including methanogens, which can increase biogas production.

Genetic engineering of methanogens: Genetic engineering is one of the most significant and advanced aspects of the modification of microbes for useful purposes. Unethical engineering techniques such as CRISPR/CAS 9 have provided a platform to modify methanogens and improve their methane production and utilization of a variety of substrates [51]. Additionally, these methanogenic strains can withstand variations in the environment and can improve the stable production of biogas in anaerobic digestion systems.

Engineering microbial community: Optimization of microbial communities and their synergistic environment can increase the production of biogas at the end of the anaerobic digestion process [52].

Carbon capture and utilization (CCU): In addition to genetic engineering technologies, the carbon capture and utilization technology is being focused on the capture of carbon dioxide that is produced in the industrial systems that are processed and converted into methane by methanogens [53]. Success in this approach can significantly increase the production of energy while decreasing the emission of greenhouse gases.

4. Factors affecting biogas production

As discussed earlier, there are various factors that can lead to an increase or decrease in the production of biogas from methanogenesis. This includes various environmental and operational factors that can collectively impact the production of biofuels, and optimization of these factors can lead to an increase in the production of methane.

4.1 Temperature

Temperature variations play a crucial role in the production of methane from methanogenic processes. These variations can affect the metabolic activity of methanogens and other microbial communities. Additionally, fluctuation in temperature beyond the optimum temperature ranges can induce a stress response and impact microbial activity, leading to a decline in methane production [54]. However, the optimum temperature range of the different classes of microbial communities in an anaerobic digestion process can vary depending upon the temperature range, that is, psychrophilic (below 20°C), mesophilic (30–40°C), and thermophilic (above 50°C) range.

The psychrophilic range is the low-temperature range in which the metabolic activity of microbes is slower in contrast to the mesophilic digestion range. This means the amount of methane produced in the process is comparatively less, however, bacteria are still able to produce methane as a byproduct [55].

The mesophilic digestion range is the most common and commercially used range in order to balance the microbial activity and stability of another big decision process [56]. The typical operating temperatures in this range are 35–37°C, and this results in efficient production of biogas.

The thermophilic temperature range is the high-temperature range that has faster degradation rates and higher production of methane, but this is an important consideration because the stability reaction process is less, and there is a high risk of microbial destruction [57]. Hence, these processes are carried out in controlled and carefully monitored environments in order to ensure maximum methane production while ensuring a lower risk (**Figure 4**).

4.2 pH levels

The variations in the pH range of the anaerobic digestion process can impact the process by affecting the enzyme activity of different metabolic enzymes and by disturbing the buffering balance of different microbial environments, which ultimately leads to fluctuating biogas production. The usual working range of methanogens is in the pH range of 6.5–8.5 [58]. The variation in the process rates, for example, a decrease in pH, can favor the acidogenesis process; however, this can offset the balance of all other steps involved in anaerobic digestion, leading to instability of the process. Additional buffer agents can be used in anaerobic digesters to increase the pH stability.

4.3 Substrate availability

The variability of substrates for the anaerobic digestion process is a crucial factor for enhancing the methanogenic activity. In addition, the utilization of waste material at the start of the process needs to be ensured to yield the maximum amount of biogas at the end of the reaction. A smooth availability of substrates means that there will be an abundance of substrates for microbial communities to consume the organic matter and convert it into useful products. Hence, to ensure maximum availability of

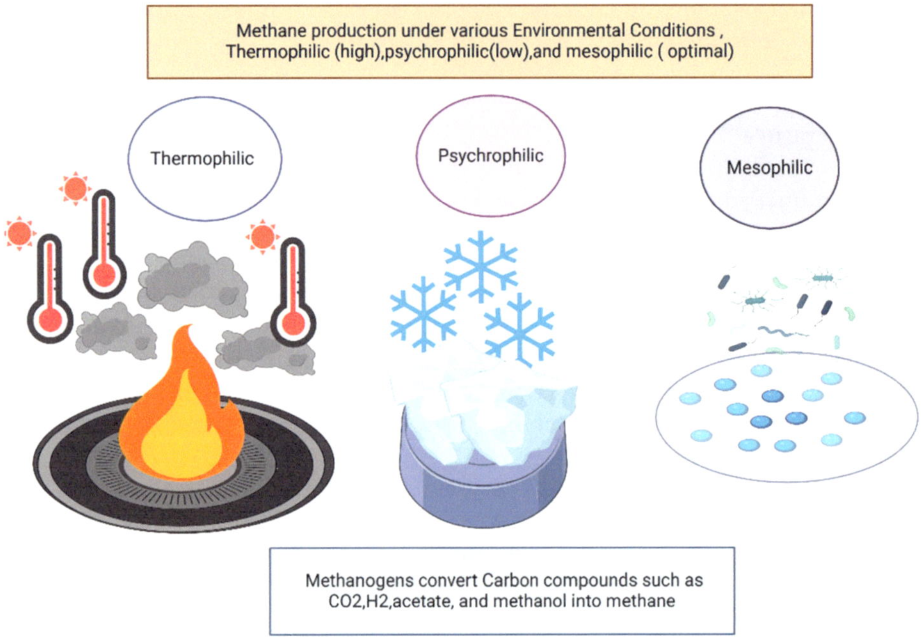

Figure 4.
Temperature ranges for methanogens growth.

substrates, various pre-treatment techniques can be applied, which include mechanical, thermal, or chemical processing to increase the surface area of the substrate for proper utilization in the anaerobic digestion process [59]. Another important factor is the proper mixing of organic waste material inside the anaerobic digestion system. Hence, the use of agitators and rotors is ensured in the anaerobic digester to ensure that there is suitable mixing and the organic material is properly exposed to microbes for maximum efficiency of biogas production. Another technique in this aspect is the co-digestion of various materials inside the bioreactor. This means that more than one type of substrate is available. This is useful as there is a diversity of microbes in the digester, and the availability of substrates means that different microbes can utilize different substrates, which leads to maximum production of biogas.

5. Innovative methanogen-based strategies

This section is focused on providing information about advanced technologies that are focused on providing key improvements for maximizing the production of biogas through anaerobic digestion.

5.1 Enhancing yields by optimizing biogas production parameters

These parameters are focused on the enhancement of the overall efficiency of anaerobic digestion to achieve maximum methane through this process:

Process monitoring and control: The crucial step of optimizing any process is to monitor the activities that are occurring in the process to optimize the fluctuating conditions and achieve a stable rate of production of desired products. In terms of biogas production, parameters such as temperature, pH, concentration of volatile fatty acids, and biogas composition are continuously monitored to achieve steady production of methane from the process [60]. This data is implemented in real time and analyzed through automated systems to have precise control over reactor conditions.

Time management for retention: Retention time means how long the process is carried out and how substrates are treated inside the reactor. Adjusting the retention time is a critical step for the optimization of the process. Parameters such as hydraulic retention time (HRT) are evaluated during reactor running to ensure that the complex organic matter is efficiently degraded into byproducts that are biodegraded to obtain biogas [61]. Longer retention times mean more degradation of organic matter and hence higher production and lower retention times mean rapid degradation rates. There is a need for balance in terms of retention times to obtain an equilibrium in the production of biogas in the process. The balance of this equilibrium also needs consideration of the choice of substrate as different feedstocks have different degradation rates and hence different hydraulic retention rates.

Pre-treatment methods: These methods comprise a set of techniques that are used to increase the substrate availability that can ensure maximum biodegradability of organic matter and hence maximum biogas yield. These methods include physical, chemical, or biological pre-treatments that can further be subcategorized [62]. However, the most common methods of pre-treatment include mechanical grinding and the freeze-thaw method, which ensure material conversion to a simpler and accessible form that can promote digestion of organic matter.

5.2 Continuous vs. batch systems

There are considerable variations between continuous and batch systems for the anaerobic digestion process that can result in different progress yields. Continuous systems allow for continuous consumption of feedstock material through input and biogas production and capture through output [63]. These systems run in a continuous fashion, and there is no interruption of the reactor operation batch systems, on the other hand are more manageable and are usually conducted at smaller-scale operation reactors. In this type of system, the processing times are longer, and the development of the products is relatively less compared to continuous batch systems. The choice between continuous and batch systems is dependent on operational goals, for how long the system is to be operated and what amounts of the product are desired.

Improved process stability: The stability of the system and reaction conditions depends on various factors and all of these factors have to be optimized to ensure that the stability of the process is achieved and there is consistency in the production of products [64]. The consideration of reactor and conditions stability is vital, as it can ensure smooth processing and desired production of biogas.

5.3 Genetic engineering of methanogens

Genetic engineering of methanogens is focused on improving the quantity of biogas produced in digesting systems by enhancing the metabolic pathways of methanogens through the implementation of genetic engineering. This leads to more efficient strains with better and diverse substrate consumption and enhanced methane production [65].

Metabolic pathway engineering: Several metabolic pathways are involved in the conversion of feedstock organic material into methane [66]. This involves a set of genes that are involved in the regulation of various parameters and conditions that lead to the activation of these pathways for biogas production. The modification of these genetic factors is a vital step that can increase the utilization of organic matter in efficient ways to get good degradation and conversion rates.

Enhancing tolerance to inhibitors: In addition to enhancing the metabolic activity of methanogens another parameter is to develop tolerance of methanogens toward several inhibitors that are produced in an anaerobic digester system. The byproducts of multiple steps involved in anaerobic digestion include ammonia and various sulfur compounds which are toxic to methanogens and can decrease their activity [67]. Hence, the modification through genetic engineering ensures that these strains have improved tolerance compared to conventional strains.

Field trials and real-world applications: The laboratory-based approaches are focused on the enhancement of methanogens, and the results hold a promise of the upgradation of methanogens. However, field trials are essential for knowing how these successful results will apply to real-world situations where there are varying environmental conditions that can affect microbes differently compared to controlled lab conditions [68].

5.4 Integration of methanogens into wastewater treatment

Methanogen integration in anaerobic environments yields biogas production. However, this reactor-based system can be combined with wastewater treatment to further enhance the process to attain certain benefits. One of such benefits is the treatment of organic matter in addition to generating renewable energy [69]. This approach can improve sustainability parameters and efficiency of wastewater treatment while ensuring steady biogas production.

Anaerobic treatment technologies: Integration of methanogens in anaerobic environments, that is, reactors, is focused on the production of biogas and its collection. Common reactor types used in this regard are anaerobic baffled reactors (ABRs) and up-flow anaerobic sludge blanket (UASB) reactors, which efficiently increase the consumption of organic matter and produce biogas [70].

Resource recovery: The additional factor for biogas production is the recovery of the amount of biogas produced followed by its processing. The end-product of digestion is slurry, which is processed waste material rich in nitrogen, phosphorus, and potassium contents. These contents can be recovered and used as excellent biofertilizers as they are in comparison to traditional fertilizers, cost-effective, efficient, and less toxic.

Decentralized treatment systems: The reactor-based systems not only provide solutions to waste management but also to the treatment of the wastewater, and this is a dual-benefit situation where waste is treated and electricity is generated simultaneously. Hence, these systems hold a promise of less greenhouse gas emissions and a positive environmental impact.

Research and development: There is ongoing research regarding the development of innovative technologies and techniques to improve anaerobic digestion for biogas production. These studies eventually aim to uplift the processing of waste material and biogas production at the same time.

6. Environmental impact and sustainability

This section focuses on emphasizing the huge potential of renewable energy systems in terms of producing a bio-based economy to provide solutions to waste management and improve energy production. There is a vast impact of these renewable energy resources, and these will produce a positive impact on several environmental and health factors indirectly which will lead to their consideration as important in comparison to other resources.

6.1 Role of methanogens in climate change mitigation

Methanogens have an important role in controlling the changes in the environment by addressing the issues of waste accumulation and greenhouse gas emissions. As this process utilizes waste materials, biogas as an energy product is produced and the slurry or end-product of digestion is used as bio-fertilizer [71].

Carbon sequestration: Anaerobic digestion system can be considered as carbon sequestration processes where greenhouse gas emissions are controlled as biogas produced is utilized as a renewable energy source [72]. This is a key point to consider when evaluating biofuels as alternatives to traditional fossil fuels.

Waste management solutions: Methanogens offer an effective solution to waste treatment technologies. In normal practice, the waste management systems used to utilize combustion for incineration and utilization of land sites for disposal of waste materials. However, in the case of anaerobic digestion, the waste materials are consumed properly and converted into useful products that are then used for various purposes.

Sustainable agriculture: The methanogens are linked to the agricultural systems in terms of the utilization of products produced in anaerobic digestion. As these products are produced after the consumption of waste, they form slurry, which serves as bio-fertilizer that is nutrient-rich fertilizer and promotes soil health.

Circular economy principles: Methanogens hold the potential to create a bio-based economy that can ensure energy production, waste management, and reduced environmental impact and climate change [73]. By conversion of organic waste into renewable energy organic waste resources are efficiently utilized.

6.2 Methanogen-driven energy systems life cycle analysis

Life cycle analysis (LCA) is an important parameter for consideration that can evaluate the environmental impact of methanogens. The life cycle of methanogens and the reactor systems is evaluated, and this can give an insight into which substrates can be utilized for energy production, which leads to improvement and sustainability [74].

Assessment of inputs and outputs: LCA helps to determine the feedstock material input for methanogenesis in anaerobic digesters. Furthermore, the outputs are also evaluated, and the comparison between input and output ratios is done to determine the balanced conditions for maximum biogas production.

Energy balance: To have an anaerobic digestion process that produces maximum biogas, LCA can help as it can determine the amount of biogas produced in relation to the amount of feedstock that is utilized. Understanding the energy balance of methanogen-driven systems is crucial for assessing their sustainability. An effective system should produce more energy in the form of biogas than is consumed in the production process. LCA can help to determine whether the energy output justifies the resources utilized, providing insights into the overall effectiveness of system.

6.3 Comparison with other renewable energy sources

In comparison to conventional energy generation systems, biogas production and utilization as an energy source are relatively more useful and offer various advantages. Insight into this comparison can help in highlighting the strengths and drawbacks of each technology and knowing which technology is most suitable depending on the amount and type of substrate available [75].

6.4 Biogas vs. solar energy

Solar energy systems transform radiations from the sun into electrical energy. In contrast, methanogens utilize organic matter for the production of biogas, which can be used for the generation of electricity. Solar energy has higher efficiency and produces more energy, but on the other hand, methanogens offer better waste management and produce energy at the same time regardless of weather conditions.

Biogas vs. wind energy: Wind energy uses energy from wind blowing across to rotate a rotor that produces electricity. Same as in the previous case, methanogens utilize organic waste and produce energy but utilize wastes and also have less environmental impact.

7. Challenges and future directions

Due to the significant use of methanogens in waste management and renewable energy, there are still some challenges that need to be addressed for better use. In this section, we investigate the technical challenges caused by methanogens, their utilization, and socioeconomic factors that restrict their widespread integration [76].

7.1 Technical challenges in methanogen utilization

Despite the optimistic potential of methanogens, there is a need to address the technical challenges that inhibit the capabilities of biogas production and environmental application:

1. Substrate variability: The proficiency of the methanogen processes is highly dependent on the substrate type and quality of the organic substrate. Different organic compounds have their own biochemical composition that impacts methane production and rate of degradation. The unstable quality of the substrate can cause fluctuations in biogas production, which results in complications in the optimization process.

2. Process stability: Anaerobic digestion is the complex chemical process that occurs in the absence of oxygen, influenced by many factors, such as PH changes, temperature fluctuations, and the collection of many inhibitory substances. The controlled environmental conditions are essential for steady biogas production any interruption can lead to less production of methane which can result in the failure of the optimistic system.

3. Inhibition by toxic compounds: The toxic compounds such as heavy metals, ammonia, and phenolic compounds that limit the activity of methanogens. Determining and reducing these inhibitors is important for healthy methanogens and enhancing the bioproduction of gas. There is a need for many advanced pre-treatment methods that decrease the toxicity of many substrates before anaerobic digestion.

4. Slow growth rates: Methanogens showed lower growth rates as compared to other microorganisms engaged in anaerobic digestion. This can inhibit the fast formation of the microbial community and lead to a longer holding time in the reactors of the biogas. This challenge can be solved by increasing the growth rates of methanogens by genetic engineering or co-culturing with the fast-growing microorganism.

5. Limited understanding of microbial interactions. The biochemical process of anaerobic digestion is associated with complex interactions among many microbial populations. There is a need for a more extensive understanding of the complex changes in the interactions among different microbial communities in order to upgrade biogas production. The advanced genomic and metagenomic techniques provide us with an understanding of microbial interaction within the methanogenic association.

6. Biogas upgrading and utilization: Many applications can be used for biogas its composition includes impurities like hydrogen sulfide and carbon dioxide, which need to be excluded for efficient use. Developing effective updating technologies is important to improve the quality of biogas and assist its incorporation in already existing energy systems.

7.2 Socioeconomic barriers

Along with many technical challenges, some socioeconomic barriers can impede the extensive implementation of methanogen-based technologies:

1. High initial investment: The capital needed to initiate methanogen-based biogas systems as a consideration, discourages the possible investors. In the long run, the cost of the functional setup may be low [77] in the developing area, primary setup and their financial needs are challenging because of the lack of resources.

2. Regulatory and policy frameworks: Irregular or unclear regulatory frameworks can create ambiguity for shareholders seeking to invest in methanogen technologies. There is a need for policymakers to create guidelines that urge shareholders to invest in the waste and energy management systems that harness methanogens, including rewards for biogas production and their implementation [78].

3. Awareness and education: In public and industrial investors, the importance and knowledge of the methanogen technologies are limited, which can hinder the implementation and acceptance of the biogas systems. Different awareness campaigns and educational programs are required in order to initiate the understanding of the importance of the methanogenic processes and their capability to contribute to long-term viability.

4. Competition with established energy sources: The energy systems that are based on methanogens may encounter competition because of the already existing energy sources like fossil fuels which are available at low costs. To support the long-term benefits of renewable energy, such as energy independence and environmental sustainability, there is a need for the implementation of methanogens technologies.

5. Community engagement: For the success of the methanogen-based projects, there is a need for local communities to be encouraged to participate in the planning and integration of these systems. For the acceptance of these technologies, it is very essential to discuss the concerns of the community and involve investors in the decision-making process to further proceed with these technologies on the road to success and stability.

7.3 Future research opportunities

To address the existing challenges of the methanogens and to increase their exploitation, many research avenues are needed to further investigate [79].

7.3.1 Advances in bioengineering

Bioengineering plays an important role in the productivity and performance of the methanogens:

1. Metabolic engineering: By utilizing different genetic engineering techniques methanogens are changed to increase the substrate utilization and improve methane. Production rates, and withstanding inhibitory compounds. The strains that are established with improved metabolic pathways can lead to better biogas production systems.

2. Synthetic biology: By using synthetic biology, enable the tailored methanogens networking, utilizing many important microbial communities in order to increase the synergistic interactions and improve biogas production. In this approach, different microbial strengths are harnessed to make a vigorous anaerobic digestion system.

3. Bioprocess optimization: Research is focused on the improved anaerobic digestion process by using the latest monitoring and control technologies. These technologies help in the increase of reliability and efficiency. The integration of real-time monitoring systems helps in the evaluation of many factors like pH, temperature, and composition of biogas that are helpful for the efficient and controlled conditions of methanogen-based biogas system productions.

7.3.2 Expanding methanogen applications

Beyond traditional biogas production techniques, the research should focus on the increasing application of methanogens:

1. Bioremediation: Examining the capability of the methanogens for bioremediation of contaminated areas, like landfills and wastewater treatment sites,

potentially creates new opportunities for the utilization of methanogens. It helps in removing toxins from organic pollutants and increases the health of the environment [80].

2. Combining renewable technologies: Analyzing the incorporation of renewable energy technologies with methanogen-based systems, like wind and solar, governs hybrid systems that increase energy production and help in the utilization of resources. This incorporation helps in the overall efficiency and durability of renewable energy systems.

3. Development of novel bioproducts: By examining the byproducts of the methanogenic processes, which are bio-fertilizers or bioplastics that increase the feasibility of the methanogen-based systems. These byproducts can seek help in the investment of stakeholders that will be helpful for the development of the system.

8. Conclusion

For environmental protection, the world is shifting toward sustainable and efficient energy resources. Methanogens play an important role in the renewable energy domain. Their capability to transform organic waste into biogas introduces environmentally friendly solutions as compared to traditional fossil fuels. They also limit the challenges of waste management and greenhouse gas emissions. In this summary section, we summarize all the key points of the methanogens that we examined, their importance in renewable energy and prospects in different fundamental domains essential for the stability of the environment.

8.1 Summary of key findings

The investigation of methanogens and their application in renewable energy unveils different interpretations:

1. Biological diversity and ecological significance: Methanogens contain diverse groups of microorganisms that have an important role in anaerobic environments, aiding substantial global carbon cycles, and impacting on changing ecosystems. The metabolic adaptability of microorganisms allows them to grow in many habitats, from wetlands to the digestive system of ruminants, leading to the balance of the ecosystem.

2. Anaerobic digestion and biogas production. The anaerobic digestion process that involves methanogens provides an effective method to transform organic waste into biogas, consisting of carbon dioxide and methane. This process plays an important role in limiting greenhouse gas emissions, organic waste disposal, and producing valuable fertilizers.

3. Innovative biotechnologies: With the advancement in biotechnology, synthetic biology and genetic engineering increases the optimization of biogas production. The innovations that play an important role in the efficiency and stability of anaerobic digestion systems, include co-digestion techniques and microbial networking.

4. Environmental impact: The climatic changes are reduced by using methanogens. They offer renewable energy solutions but instead depend on fossil fuels. The methanogen-based energy system attains the reduction of greenhouse gas emissions as compared to conventional energy sources.

5. Challenges and barriers: Methanogens have great capabilities and high adaptation in anaerobic conditions, still there are many challenges in the integration of methanogens-based systems, including technical hurdles, required vigorous regulatory frameworks, and socioeconomic barriers. To reduce these challenges, there is a need for continuous efforts by researchers, policymakers, and industry investors.

8.2 The future role of methanogens in renewable energy

Methanogens are an important contributor to substantial energy systems because of their ability to transform a variety of organic waste materials into renewable energy sources. This capability is helpful for the ecosystem and limits carbon emissions and waste. There are many trends that are important to shape the future of methanogens and their role in sustainability.

1. Integration with circular economy: Economic models are changed and shifted rounds, according to the needs of society. Methanogens are essential transitions of recycling organic waste material into the products that are valuable and sustainable. The integration of these methanogens into systems is not only helpful for efficient resources but also supports the best waste management practices.

2. Collaboration with renewable energy systems: The role of methanogens is enhanced by combining these technologies with other systems. Examples of these synergistic systems are solar and wind which provide a continuous and stable energy source. The multiple sources combine and form a hybrid, this hybrid is essential for efficient energy reliability and security.

3. Advancements in research and development: The research that is continuously focused on methanogens, their microbial interactions, and metabolic pathways, leads to innovation in biogas technologies. Due to the discovery of new technologies, the bioengineering of the methanogen base system is improved which enhances the production of biogas. The improved methanogen base system is more economical than conventional systems because of the efficient production.

4. Policy support and incentives: To increase the capability of methanogens in renewable energy it is important to make strict guidelines for supporting renewable sources. Different government and regulatory bodies play an important role in endorsing public awareness about the importance of methanogen base systems and support financially through industry investors.

5. Global collaboration: Climatic change is a global problem. Methanogen-based systems are eco-friendly and best for a healthy environment. It is essential for the collective efforts of researchers, industry leaders, and the government to share the resources and knowledge that are helpful for the development of methanogen-based solutions worldwide.

Conflict of interest

The authors declare no conflict of interest.

Author details

Muhammad Junaid Ahmad Tariq[1*], Jasia Javed[1], Ume Habiba[1] and Sameen Meer[2]

1 Pak-Austria Fachhochschule Institute of Applied Sciences and Technology, Haripur, Pakistan

2 Edinburgh Napier University, Edinburgh, United Kingdom

*Address all correspondence to: junaidtariq186@gmail.com

References

[1] Growth and survival of anaerobic fungi in batch culture and in the digestive tract of ruminants - ProQuest [Internet]. Available from: https://www.proquest.com/openview/4bfbaa0df72039bad23be47878785019/1?pq-origsite=gscholar&cbl=2026366&diss=y [Accessed: October 21, 2024]

[2] Biogas as a sustainable energy source for developing countries: Opportunities and challenges [Internet]. Available from: https://www.infona.pl/resource/bwmeta1.element.elsevier-e8c5e74e-eb99-3bcb-b63c-b5944fd933de [Accessed: October 21, 2024]

[3] Energy, Environment and Sustainable Development. Nottingham, UK: ScienceDirect [Internet]; 2007. Available from: https://www.sciencedirect.com/science/article/abs/pii/S1364032107000834; [Accessed: October 21, 2024]

[4] Mac Kinnon MA, Brouwer J, Samuelsen S. The role of natural gas and its infrastructure in mitigating greenhouse gas emissions, improving regional air quality, and renewable resource integration. Progress in Energy and Combustion Science. 2018;**64**:62-92

[5] Policy instruments for environmental and natural resource management – [Internet]. Available from: https://www.taylorfrancis.com/books/mono/10.4324/9781315780894/policy-instruments-environmental-natural-resource-management-jessica-coria-thomas-sterner [Accessed: October 21, 2024]

[6] Clark DS, Ludlow JM, Nelson CM, Shah NN, Miller JF. Pressure and temperature effects on growth and methane production of the extreme thermophile Methanococcus jannaschii. Applied and Environmental Microbiology [Internet]. 12 Dec 1988;**54**. DOI: 10.1128/aem.54.12.3039-3042.1988

[7] Gaby JC, Zamanzadeh M, Horn SJ. The effect of temperature and retention time on methane production and microbial community composition in staged anaerobic digesters fed with food waste. Biotechnology for Biofuels. 2017;**10**(1):302

[8] Mah RA. Methanogenesis and methanogenic partnerships. Philosophical Transactions of the Royal Society of London. B, Biological Sciences [Internet]. School of Public Health, University of California, Los Angeles, California, USA. 11 Jun 1982. DOI: 10.1098/rstb.1982.0064 [Accessed: October 21, 2024]

[9] Li Y, Chen Y, Wu J. Enhancement of methane production in anaerobic digestion process: A review. Applied Energy. 2019;**240**:120-137

[10] Ziemiński K, Frąc M. Methane fermentation process as anaerobic digestion of biomass: Transformations, stages and microorganisms. African Journal of Biotechnology. 2012;**11**(18):4127-4139

[11] Omer AM. Energy use and environmental impacts: A general review. Journal of Renewable and Sustainable Energy. 2009;**1**(5):053101

[12] Omer AM. Green energies and the environment. Renewable and Sustainable Energy Reviews. 2008;**12**(7):1789-1821

[13] Tester JW, Drake EM, Driscoll MJ, Golay MW, Peters WA. Sustainable energy. In: Choosing Among Options. 2nd ed. Google Books [Internet].

Cambridge, Massachusetts: MIT Press; 2012. Available from: https://books.google.com.pk/books?hl=en&lr=&id=pd7xCwAAQBAJ&oi=fnd&pg=PR5&dq=The+utilization+of+sustainable+energy+alternatives+is+however+an+alternative+approach+to+address+all+these+issues+and+to+produce+a+renewable+form+of+energy+that+can+be+utilized+in+a+renewable+way&ots=UQToBH8-Po&sig=CQvCr9E2OoYWTRk7ym-LRpe8eTA&redir_esc=y#v=onepage&q&f=false; [Accessed: October 21, 2024]

[14] Shaji H, Chandran V, Mathew L. Chapter 13 - organic fertilizers as a route to controlled release of nutrients. In: Lewu FB, Volova T, Thomas S, Rakhimol RK, editors. Controlled Release Fertilizers for Sustainable Agriculture [Internet]. School of Biosciences, Mahatma Gandhi University, Kottayam, Kerala, India: Academic Press; 2021. pp. 231-245. Available from: https://www.sciencedirect.com/science/article/pii/B9780128195550000133 [Accessed: October 21, 2024]

[15] Kumar S, Shrestha P, Abdul SP. A review of biofuel policies in the major biofuel producing countries of ASEAN: Production, targets, policy drivers and impacts. Renewable and Sustainable Energy Reviews. 2013;**26**:822-836

[16] Silverman RE, Flores RJ, Brouwer J. Energy and economic assessment of distributed renewable gas and electricity generation in a small disadvantaged urban community. Applied Energy. 2020;**280**:115974

[17] Thirunavukkarasu M, Sawle Y, Lala H. A Comprehensive Review on Optimization of Hybrid Renewable Energy Systems Using Various Optimization Techniques. ScienceDirect [Internet]. Vellore, India: VIT University; 2023. Available from: https://www.sciencedirect.com/science/article/abs/pii/S1364032123000485; [Accessed: October 21, 2024]

[18] Amin FR, Khalid H, El-Mashad HM, Chen C, Liu G, Zhang R. Functions of bacteria and archaea participating in the bioconversion of organic waste for methane production. The Science of the Total Environment. 2021;**763**:143007

[19] Garcia-Peña EI, Parameswaran P, Kang DW, Canul-Chan M, Krajmalnik-Brown R. Anaerobic Digestion and co-Digestion Processes of Vegetable and Fruit Residues: Process and Microbial Ecology. Mexico City, Mexico: ScienceDirect [Internet]; 2011. Available from: https://www.sciencedirect.com/science/article/abs/pii/S0960852411010194; [Accessed: October 21, 2024]

[20] Boone DR, Whitman WB, Rouvière P. Diversity and taxonomy of methanogens. In: Ferry JG, editor. Methanogenesis: Ecology, Physiology, Biochemistry & Genetics [Internet]. Boston, MA: Springer US; 1993. pp. 35-80. DOI: 10.1007/978-1-4615-2391-8_2 [Accessed: October 21, 2024]

[21] Buan NR. Methanogens: Pushing the boundaries of biology. Emerging Topics in Life Sciences. 2018;**2**(4): 629-646

[22] Archaeal clusters of orthologous genes (arCOGs): An update and application for analysis of shared features between thermococcales, methanococcales, and methanobacteriales [Internet]. Available from: https://www.mdpi.com/2075-1729/5/1/818 [Accessed: October 21, 2024]

[23] Baptiste E, Brochier C, Boucher Y. Higher-Level Classification of the Archaea: Evolution of Methanogenesis and Methanogens – Bapteste – Archaea. Wiley Online Library [Internet]. Victoria,

Canada: Heron Publishing; 2005. DOI: 10.1155/2005/859728 [Accessed: October 21, 2024]

[24] Gene order phylogeny and the evolution of methanogens. PLoS One [Internet]. Available from: https://journals.plos.org/plosone/article?id=10.1371/journal.pone.0006069. [Accessed: October 21, 2024]

[25] Fardeau ML, Cayol JL, Ollivier B. Methanocalculus. In: Bergey's Manual of Systematics of Archaea and Bacteria (BMSAB) [Internet]. Hoboken, New Jersey, USA: John Wiley & Sons, Inc; 2019. Available from: https://hal.science/hal-02883889 [Accessed: October 21, 2024]

[26] Kurth JM, Huub J. Op den Camp M, Welte CU. Several ways one goal—Methanogenesis from unconventional substrates. Applied Microbiology and Biotechnology [Internet]. 2020;**104**:6839-6854. Available from:. DOI: 10.1007/s00253-020-10724-7 [Accessed: October 21, 2024]

[27] Ferry JG. The chemical biology of methanogenesis. Planetary and Space Science. 2010;**58**(14):1775-1783

[28] Lei Lv, Serge Maurice Mbadinga, Li-Ying Wang, Jin-Feng Liu, Ji-Dong Gu, Bo-Zhong Mu, Shi-Zhong Yang. Acetoclastic methanogenesis is likely the dominant biochemical pathway of palmitate degradation in the presence of sulfate. Applied Microbiology and Biotechnology [Internet]. 2015;**99**:7757-7769. DOI: 10.1007/s00253-015-6669-z [Accessed: October 21, 2024]

[29] Large PJ. Methylotrophy and Methanogenesis. Google Books [Internet]. American Society for Microbiology. Original from the University of Michigan Digitized 2 Mar 2010. 1983. Available from: https://books.google.com.pk/books?hl=en&lr=&id=iIHtCAAAQBAJ&oi=fnd&pg=PA1&dq=Classification+of+Methanogenesis+pathways+Methylotrophic+Methanogenesis&ots=o5WmBX72Kd&sig=olSTJlaVcBGuaAzXPTKxdmK-MjE&redir_esc=y#v=onepage&q=Classification%20of%20Methanogenesis%20pathways%20Methylotrophic%20Methanogenesis&f=false; [Accessed: October 21, 2024]

[30] Lyu Z, Lu Y. Metabolic shift at the class level sheds light on adaptation of methanogens to oxidative environments. The ISME Journal [Internet]. Feb 2018;**12**(2):411-423. DOI: 10.1038/ismej.2017.173. Published: 14 November 2017 [Accessed: October 21, 2024]

[31] Ma Y, Qu Y, Yao X, Xia C, Lv M, Lin X, et al. Unveiling the unique role of iron in the metabolism of methanogens: A review. Environmental Research. 2024;**250**:118495

[32] Zabranska J, Pokorna D. Bioconversion of carbon dioxide to methane using hydrogen and hydrogenotrophic methanogens. Biotechnology Advances. 2018;**36**(3):707-720

[33] Contreras G, Thomsen J, Pfitzer M, Hafenbradl D, Kostner D, Holtmann D, et al. New perspectives for biotechnological applications of methanogens. Current Research in Biotechnology. 2022;**4**:468-474

[34] van Leeuwenhoek A. Methanogenesis in Thermophilic Biogas Reactors [Internet]. DOI: 10.1007/BF00872197

[35] Role of Microbial Hydrolysis in Anaerobic Digestion [Internet]. Available from: https://www.mdpi.com/1996-1073/13/21/5555 [Accessed: October 21, 2024]

[36] Frontiers. Hydrolysis and Methanogenesis in UASB-AnMBR Treating Municipal Wastewater under Psychrophilic Conditions: Importance of Reactor Configuration and Inoculum [Internet]. DOI: 10.3389/fbioe.2020.567695/full [Accessed: October 21, 2024]

[37] Huang W, Wang Z, Zhou Y, Ng WJ. The role of hydrogenotrophic methanogens in an acidogenic reactor. Chemosphere. 2015;**140**:40-46

[38] Taconi KA, Zappi ME, Todd French W, Brown LR. Methanogenesis under acidic pH conditions in a semi-continuous reactor system. Bioresource Technology. 2008;**99**(17):8075-8081

[39] Kim. Kinetics of acetogenesis and methanogenesis in anaerobic reactions under toxic conditions. Water Environment Research [Internet]. 1994. DOI: 10.2175/WER.66.2.5 [Accessed: October 21, 2024]

[40] Venkata Mohan S, Mohanakrishna G, Sarma PN. Integration of acidogenic and methanogenic processes for simultaneous production of biohydrogen and methane from wastewater treatment. International Journal of Hydrogen Energy. 2008;**33**(9):2156-2166

[41] Tg I, Haq I, Kalamdhad AS. 14 - Factors affecting anaerobic digestion for biogas production: A review. In: Hussain C, Hait S, editors. Advanced Organic Waste Management [Internet]. Department of Civil Engineering, Indian Institute of Technology, Guwahati, Assam, India. 2022. pp. 223-233. Available from: https://www.sciencedirect.com/science/article/pii/B9780323857925000204 [Accessed: October 21, 2024]

[42] Cho YT, Young JC; Jordan JA, Moon HM. Factors affecting measurement of specific methanogenic activity. Water Science & Technology [Internet] Vol. 52. Available from: https://iwaponline.com/wst/article-abstract/52/1-2/435/13007/Factors-affecting-measurement-of-specific. [Accessed: October 21, 2024]

[43] Samir Kumar Khanal. Anaerobic Biotechnology for Bioenergy Production. Wiley Online Books [Internet]; Iowa State University in the United States. First published: 26 September 2008. DOI: 10.1002/9780813804545#page=103 [Accessed: October 21, 2024]

[44] Yamasaki R, Maeda T, Wood TK. Electron carriers increase electricity production in methane microbial fuel cells that reverse methanogenesis. Biotechnology for Biofuels and Bioproducts [Internet]. 2018;**11**:211, p. 10. Published: 25 July 2018. DOI: 10.1186/s13068-018-1208-7 [Accessed: October 21, 2024]

[45] Vilela RS, Fuess LT, Saia FT, Silveira CRM, Oliveira CA, Andrade PA, et al. Biofuel production from sugarcane molasses in thermophilic anaerobic structured-bed reactors. Renewable and Sustainable Energy Reviews. 2021;**144**:110974

[46] Burkhardt M, Jordan I, Heinrich S, Behrens J, Ziesche A, Busch G. Long term and demand-oriented biocatalytic synthesis of highly concentrated methane in a trickle bed reactor. Applied Energy. 2019;**240**:818-826

[47] Yang Z, Wang W, He Y, Zhang R, Liu G. Effect of ammonia on methane production, methanogenesis pathway, microbial community and reactor performance under mesophilic and thermophilic conditions. Renewable Energy. 2018;**125**:915-925

[48] Herrmann C, Ramm P, Murphy JD. The relationship between bioreactor

design and feedstock for optimal biogas production. In: Liao Q, Shu CJ, Herrmann C, Xia A, editors. Bioreactors for Microbial Biomass and Energy Conversion [Internet]. Singapore: Springer; 2018. pp. 163-197. DOI: 10.1007/978-981-10-7677-0_5 [Accessed: October 21, 2024]

[49] Pandya RS, Kaur T, Bhattacharya R, Bose D, Saraf D. Harnessing microorganisms for bioenergy with microbial fuel cells: Powering the future. Water-Energy Nexus. 2024;**7**:1-12

[50] Nguyen LN, Kumar J, Vu MT, Mohammed JAH, Pathak N, Commault AS, et al. Biomethane production from anaerobic co-digestion at wastewater treatment plants: A critical review on development and innovations in biogas upgrading techniques. Science of The Total Environment. 2021;**765**:142753

[51] Myers T, Dykstra CM. Teaching old dogs new tricks: Genetic engineering methanogens. Applied and Environmental Microbiology [Internet]. 10 Jun 2024;**90**(7):17. DOI: 10.1128/aem.02247-23 [Accessed: October 21, 2024]

[52] Dykstra CM, Pavlostathis SG. Methanogenic biocathode microbial community development and the role of bacteria. Environmental Science & Technology [Internet]. 3 Apr 2017;**51**(9):20. DOI: 10.1021/acs.est.6b04112 [Accessed: October 21, 2024]

[53] Wu L, Hou Z, Xie Y, Luo Z, Huang L, Wu X, et al. Carbon capture, circular utilization, and sequestration (CCCUS): A multifunctional technology coupling underground biomethanation with geothermal energy production. Journal of Cleaner Production. 2023;**426**:139225

[54] Demollari E, Jojic E, Vorpsi V, Dodona E, Sallaku E. Temperature and stirring effect of biogas production from two different systems. American Journal of Energy Engineering. 2017;**5**(4):6-10

[55] Tiwari BR, Rouissi T, Brar SK, Surampalli RY. Critical insights into psychrophilic anaerobic digestion: Novel strategies for improving biogas production. Waste Management. 2021;**131**:513-526

[56] The comparison of mesophilic and thermophilic anaerobic digestion - Document - Gale Academic OneFile [Internet]. Available from: https://go.gale.com/ps/i.do?id=GALE%7CA224335535&sid=googleScholar&v=2.1&it=r&linkaccess=abs&issn=17269687&p=AONE&sw=w&userGroupName=anon%7Eed83e8e1&aty=open-web-entry [Accessed: October 21, 2024]

[57] Zinder SH, Anguish T, Cardwell SC. Effects of temperature on methanogenesis in a thermophilic (58°C) anaerobic digestor. Applied and Environmental Microbiology [Internet]. 1984;**47**:4. DOI: 10.1128/aem.47.4.808-813.1984 [Accessed: October 21, 2024]

[58] Fang LC, Zhong YX, Ming ZG, Wei LW, Li J. Prediction of methane yield at optimum pH for anaerobic digestion of organic fraction of municipal solid waste. Bioresource Technology. 2008;**99**(4):882-888

[59] Basic Principles of Bioconversions in Anaerobic Digestion and Methanogenesis. SpringerLink [Internet]. DOI: 10.1007/978-1-4757-0301-6_15 [Accessed: October 22, 2024]

[60] Sarker S, Lamb JJ, Hjelme DR, Lien KM. A review of the role of critical parameters in the design and operation of biogas production plants. Applied Sciences. 2019;**9**(9):1915

[61] Kuruti K, Begum S, Ahuja S, Anupoju GR, Juntupally S, Gandu B,

et al. Exploitation of rapid acidification phenomena of food waste in reducing the hydraulic retention time (HRT) of high rate anaerobic digester without conceding on biogas yield. Bioresource Technology. 2017;**226**:65-72

[62] Zeb I, Yousaf S, Ali M, Yasmeen A, Khan AZ, Tariq JA, et al. *In-situ* microaeration of anaerobic digester treating buffalo manure for enhanced biogas yield. Renewable Energy. 2022;**181**:843-850

[63] Comparative evaluation of batch and continuous process biogas production from animal wastes. International Journal of Ambient Energy;**37**(1) [Internet]. DOI: 10.1080/01430750.2013.874369 [Accessed: October 22, 2024]

[64] Chen C, Guo W, Ngo HH, Lee DJ, Tung KL, Jin P, et al. Challenges in biogas production from anaerobic membrane bioreactors. Renewable Energy. 2016;**98**:120-134

[65] Enzmann F, Mayer F, Rothe M, Holtmann D. Methanogens: Biochemical Background and Biotechnological Applications. AMB Express [Internet]. 2018. DOI: 10.1186/S13568-017-0531-X [Accessed: October 22, 2024]

[66] Majidian P, Tabatabaei M, Zeinolabedini M, Naghshbandi MP, Chisti Y. Metabolic Engineering of Microorganisms for Biofuel Production. ScienceDirect [Internet]. Agricultural Biotechnology Research Institute of Iran (ABRII), Agricultural Research, Education and Extension Organization (AREEO), Karaj, Iran. 2016. Available from: https://www.sciencedirect.com/science/article/abs/pii/S1364032117314636; [Accessed: October 22, 2024]

[67] Wikandari R, Sanjaya AP, Millati R, Karimi K, Taherzadeh MJ. Chapter 20 - Fermentation inhibitors in ethanol and biogas processes and strategies to counteract their effects. In: Pandey A, Larroche C, Dussap CG, Gnansounou E, Khanal SK, Ricke S, editors. Biofuels: Alternative Feedstocks and Conversion Processes for the Production of Liquid and Gaseous Biofuels, Biomass, Biofuels, Biochemicals. Department of Food and Agricultural Product Technology, Universitas Gadjah Mada, Yogyakarta, Indonesia. Available from: https://www.sciencedirect.com/science/article/pii/B9780128168561000208. 2nd ed Edition) [Internet]. Academic Press; 2019. pp. 461-499 [Accessed: October 22, 2024]

[68] Lichtman R, Ellegård A, Lal S, Sharma N. The improved biogas systems project: Results and future work. Energy for Sustainable Development. 1996;**3**(4):28-42

[69] Lettinga G. Sustainable integrated biological wastewater treatment. Water Science and Technology. 1996;**33**(3):85-98

[70] Mara D, Horan NJ. Handbook of Water and Wastewater Microbiology. School of civil engineering, University of leeds, UK. Elsevier; 2003. 828 p

[71] Chew KR, Leong HY, Khoo KS, Vo DVN, Anjum H, Chang CK, et al. Effects of anaerobic digestion of food waste on biogas production and environmental impacts: A review. Environmental Chemistry Letters. 2021;**19**(4):2921-2939

[72] Mohd Yasin NH, Maeda T, Hu A, Yu CP, Wood TK. CO_2 sequestration by methanogens in activated sludge for methane production. Applied Energy. 2015;**142**:426-434

[73] Ellacuriaga M, García-Cascallana J, Gómez X. Biogas production from organic

wastes: Integrating concepts of circular economy. Fuels. 2021;**2**(2):144-167

[74] Zhang T, Tremblay PL. Chapter 5.6 - Possible industrial applications for microbial electrosynthesis from carbon dioxide. In: Mohan SV, Varjani S, Pandey A, editors. Microbial Electrochemical Technology [Internet], Biomass, Biofuels and Biochemicals. Engineering and Life Science, Wuhan University of Technology, Wuhan, People's Republic of China. Available from: https://www.sciencedirect.com/science/article/pii/B9780444640529000340. Elsevier; 2019. pp. 825-842 [Accessed: October 22, 2024]

[75] Mignogna D, Ceci P, Cafaro C, Corazzi G, Avino P. Production of biogas and biomethane as renewable energy sources: A review. Applied Sciences. 2023;**13**(18):10219

[76] Beauchemin KA, Ungerfeld EM, Eckard RJ, Wang M. Review: Fifty years of research on rumen methanogenesis: Lessons learned and future challenges for mitigation. Animal [Internet] Vol. 14. Issue S1. Available from: https://www.cambridge.org/core/journals/animal/article/review-fifty-years-of-research-on-rumen-methanogenesis-lessons-learned-and-future-challenges-for-mitigation/8F7537B81CBDA633F48663C1ACF33036#. [Accessed: October 22, 2024]

[77] Roopnarain A, Ndaba B, Bello-Akinosho M, Bamuza-Pemu E, Mukhuba M, Nkuna R, et al. Biogas Technology in Africa: An assessment of feedstock, barriers, socio-economic impact and the way forward. In: Balagurusamy N, Chandel AK, editors. Biogas Production: From Anaerobic Digestion to a Sustainable Bioenergy Industry [Internet]. Cham: Springer International Publishing; 2020. pp. 415-445. DOI: 10.1007/978-3-030-58827-4_18 [Accessed: October 22, 2024]

[78] Abanades S, Abbaspour H, Ahmadi A, Das B, Ehyaei MA, Esmaeilion F, et al. A critical review of biogas production and usage with legislations framework across the globe. International Journal of Environmental Science and Technology [Internet]. 2022;**19**:3377-3400. Published: 16 May 2021. DOI: 10.1007/s13762-021-03301-6 [Accessed: October 22, 2024]

[79] Frontiers. Evolving understanding of rumen methanogen ecophysiology [Internet]. Available from: https://www.frontiersin.org/journals/microbiology/articles/10.3389/fmicb.2023.1296008/full [Accessed: October 22, 2024]

[80] Ray S, Kuppam C, Pandit S, Kumar P. Biogas upgrading by hydrogenotrophic methanogens: An overview. Waste and Biomass Valorization. 2023;**14**(2):537-552

Chapter 3

Genomic Mobility: Transposons in Methanoarchaea

Luise Rentz, Finn O. Gehlert and Ruth A. Schmitz

Abstract

Methanoarchaea, a unique group of archaea, play a crucial role in the global carbon cycle through methanogenesis, a process where different carbon sources such as carbon dioxide (CO_2)/hydrogen (H_2), acetate, formate, methanol, and methylamines are metabolized and methane is produced. Transposons are mobile genetic elements (MGEs) capable of moving within and between genomes, thus significantly influencing genetic diversity and evolution. This chapter will investigate the presence, diversity, and functional implications of transposons in methanoarchaea. We explore the various types of transposable elements (TEs) identified in methanogenic genomes and highlight their structural and functional characteristics. Our focus is on insertion sequences (IS), miniature inverted-repeat transposable elements (MITEs), and the recently described casposons, which show similarities to eukaryotic transposons, using Cas1 solo as the transposase. Summarizing current knowledge on the diversity, mechanisms, and impacts of TEs in methanoarchaea reveals their significant role in genome plasticity, adaptation to diverse environmental conditions, and potential contributions to horizontal gene transfer (HGT) within microbial communities. Understanding transposons in methanoarchaea not only provides insight into the fundamental processes governing microbial evolution but also offers potential applications in biotechnology and environmental management. This review synthesizes current understanding of archaeal TEs, focusing on their diversity, mechanisms, and evolutionary significance.

Keywords: mobile genetic elements (MGEs), transposons, insertion sequences (IS), miniature inverted-repeat transposable elements (MITEs), casposons, methanoarchaea, CRISPR-Cas systems, Cas1 solo, genome evolution

1. Introduction

Mobile genetic elements (MGEs) are key players in the dynamic landscape of genomes, contributing significantly to genetic diversity, evolution, and adaptation across various organisms and are further exchanged via horizontal gene transfer (HGT) [1, 2]. MGEs include various elements, such as viruses, plasmids, and transposons, that can shift their genomic position within a host or between host cells [1, 2]. MGEs are DNA sequences capable of moving or copying themselves to new positions within a genome of a single cell (intracellular translocation) or transferring between two or more cells (HGT). In addition to the core genes necessary for transfer, MGEs

 IntechOpen

often carry accessory genes that provide selective advantages (e.g., resistances). Furthermore, the rearrangement due to MGEs plays a crucial role in genome evolution, adaptation, and variability as they can disrupt existing genes, create new gene combinations, or alter gene expression, leading to significant shifts in the host organism's phenotype. MGEs in archaea are less extensively studied compared to those in bacteria and eukaryotes. The limited knowledge of MGEs in archaea arises from the challenges associated with the complex isolation and cultivation methods required for those organisms. Especially the more unique and outstanding properties of archaea, often inhabiting some of the most extreme environments on Earth, rely heavily on the mutational benefits of MGEs. The transfer of genes between species is one of the most powerful strategies to adapt and survive under those harsh conditions. Studies have shown that MGEs in archaea contribute to their genetic diversity and ability to thrive in extreme conditions by transferring genes crucial for survival and adaptation. The distribution of MGEs varies inside the archaeal domain, with notable prevalence in extremophiles [3–5]. In particular, the *Halobacteriales*, *Sulfolobales*, *Thermoplasmatales*, and *Methanosarcinales* often harbor a rich variety of MGEs [3, 6–8]. For this review, we are mainly focusing on the specialized group of *Methanoarchaea*, *Sulfolobales,* and *Halobacteriales*. Due to their methane production, these microorganisms are vital to the carbon cycle. Further, we will focus on the group of transposable elements and will in detail summarize the knowledge on the recently described prominent casposons found exclusively in archaea.

2. Main

2.1 Mobile genetic elements in general

Mobile genetic elements occur in all three domains of life and include transposons, plasmids, and viruses (**Figure 1**). *Viruses and phages* possess linear or circular genomes of single- or double-stranded DNA or RNA, which are typically encapsulated in protein and lipid membranes. In some cases, they display mechanistic or structural similarities to plasmids and transposons [10–13]. Another prominent class of MGEs are *plasmids* which are small, circular DNA molecules that can replicate independently in prokaryotic cells, often carrying genes that provide selective advantages such as antibiotic resistance (resistance plasmids) [10]. While conjugative plasmids are able to transfer between prokaryotes via conjugation, non-conjugative plasmids are immobile [14, 15]. Besides resistance plasmids, some cells exhibit degradative plasmids that contain genes that enable the host cell to metabolize unfamiliar substrates. Pointing out archaea, for example, the plasmid pDLI0 in *Desulfurolobus ambivalens* harbors genes involved in sulfur metabolism, enabling the archaeon to utilize sulfur compounds as energy sources and adapt to extreme environments [16]. The plasmid *pTIK4*, found in the crenarchaeal thermoacidophile strain *Sulfolobus neozealandicus*, enables its host to outcompete or eliminate rival *Sulfolobus* strains without the need to diffuse a toxic agent, potentially through cell contact [17].

One of the most well-studied types of MGEs is *transposons* that can change their position within the genome, causing mutations and altering the cell's genetic identity. These "jumping genes", first discovered by Barbara McClintock in maize plants in the 1940s, play a significant role in genome evolution and diversity [18–20]. Nowadays transposons are known to be ubiquitous across all life forms, including archaea [3, 21, 22]. Some transposons can exhibit an extrachromosomal stage resembling

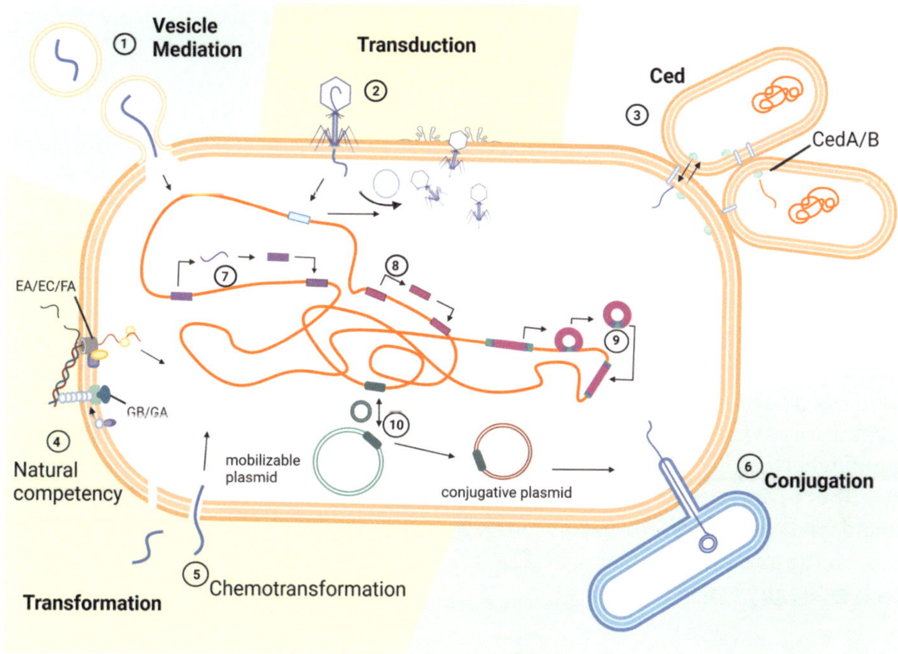

Figure 1.
Horizontal Gene Transfer Mechanisms. The diagram illustrates multiple mechanisms for DNA uptake or exchange in prokaryotic cells as well as intracellular processes that show mobile genetic elements: (1) Vesicle-mediated transformation involves DNA delivery via vesicles. (2) Transduction involves the transfer of viral DNA into a host cell via phages. (3) Ced as a crenarchaeal system for exchange of DNA that occurs in Sulfolobus *strains. Transformation can be (4) natural, with naturally competent cells taking up free DNA from the environment (e.g.,* B. subtilis*), or (5) induced in the laboratory, through e.g., chemotransformation. (6) Conjugation occurs through direct DNA transfer between cells mediated by a conjugative pilus. (7) Retrotransposons move via an RNA intermediate in a "copy-and-paste" mechanism, facilitated by transposase enzymes. (8) DNA Transposons move mainly via an "cut-and-paste" mechanism but also can use a "copy-and-paste" mechanism. (9) Caspsons, exclusively found in archaea, move via a distinct mechanism where a loop-structure is formed prior to excision from its original target site leaving an empty target site left in the genome and a circular intermediate of the casposon. (10) Transposons integrate into new sites on the chromosome or plasmids by non-homologous recombination (adapted from [9], created in BioRender.com.).*

plasmids [23–25]. These transposons, whether encoded on chromosomes or extra-chromosomal DNA, can be transferred between cells via phages or plasmids [10, 14, 26]. Transposons can be autonomous, carrying the necessary genes for their own transposition, or non-autonomous, requiring enzymes encoded by other elements for movement [27, 28]. Additionally, transposons may sometimes carry intact or defective segments of phage capsid proteins [29, 30]. The detection of a wide variety of transposons required a practical classification system, resulting in transposons being primarily categorized by their translocation mechanisms as well as their size, structure, gene organization, and domain structure of their encoded proteins [27, 31, 32].

At first, transposons are classified into two main categories based on their transposition mechanisms: Class I (retrotransposons) move via an RNA intermediate in a "copy-and-paste" mechanism. In this process, the transposon is first transcribed into RNA, which is then reverse-transcribed back into DNA by reverse transcriptase and inserted into a new location in the genome mediated by integrases [27, 28, 33]. On the other hand, Class II (DNA transposons) primarily utilize a "cut-and-paste" mechanism that is facilitated by transposase enzymes. In this mechanism, the transposon is excised from its original location and integrated into a new site within the genome. Although Class II transposons predominantly operate through the "cut-and-paste" mechanism, some may exhibit a "copy-and-paste" mechanism [27, 28, 33]. Most DNA transposons are characterized by terminal inverted repeats (TIRs) and their linear structure and include families like Tc1–Mariner and Transib belonging to subclass 1, and Mavericks belonging to subclass 2 [27, 34, 35].

Retrotransposons further subdivide into long terminal repeat (LTR) retrotransposons, which have repeated sequences at both ends and non-LTR retrotransposons, which lack these repeats [28, 36, 37]. LTR retrotransposons are particularly abundant in many eukaryotes, such as flowering plants, animals, and yeasts [37–40].

In summary, MGEs are fundamental to genetic diversity and evolution. Their ability to move and integrate across different genomic contexts plays an important role in shaping genomes, influencing evolutionary processes, and driving the adaptation of organisms to changing environments. The detailed classification of transposons, beyond whether they use an RNA intermediate, varies widely among publications and author groups, remaining a topic of active debate and continual evolution as new transposon types are discovered [32, 41]. However, most of these classifications were based on the analysis of eukaryotic TEs, and their relevance to prokaryotic transposons is generally restricted [32, 41].

2.2 Intercellular transfer mechanisms in archaea

Although transduction, conjugation, and transformation (**Figure 1**) have been initially discovered for bacteria, several have been also identified in a small number of archaeal species [14]. Transduction is a process of MGE transfer mediated by viruses and is divided into undirected general transduction which includes lytic and lysogenic phages and specialized transduction which includes only lysogenic phages [42–45]. Lytic phages cause rapid lysis of the host cells, immediately starting to replicate and thereby releasing new phages. In contrast, lysogenic phages integrate their genome into the host cell's chromosome or maintain it as an extra-chromosomal element known as a prophage, resulting in an inactive state that is replicated alongside the host's DNA during cell division [14, 42]. In this state, some genes may be expressed, which can provide advantages to the host, such as immunity to superinfection by other phages. For example, the *cI* gene of the Lambda Phage encodes the lambda repressor protein, which maintains the prophage state by inhibiting the activation of the lytic cycle [46]. Lysogenic phages can switch between the lysogenic lifestyle, where they remain integrated, and the lytic lifestyle, where they activate and begin replicating. This switch is influenced by environmental conditions and the general infection state within the host cell population using quorum sensing-like mechanisms [47, 48].

While transduction is extensively studied in bacteria, this phenomenon has also been observed in various archaeal environments [49]. Since the first discovery of archaeal viruses infecting *Halobacterium salinarium* in 1974, genome sequencing has uncovered a wide variety of proviruses within archaeal genomes [49–51]. Studies have shown that archaeal viruses can package host DNA during proliferation and amplification and subsequently introduce this genetic material into new host cells [52–54]. Research has documented the role of Sulfolobus spindle-shaped viruses (SSVs) in the transfer of host genes among *Sulfolobus* species, highlighting the significance of viral-mediated gene transfer in archaeal evolution and ecology [49, 54].

In contrast, conjugation involves the direct transfer of genetic material between cells through physical contact and is dependent on autonomously replicating elements like chromosomally integrated conjugative elements (ICEs), conjugative transposons (CTns) or conjugative plasmids. This process has been observed in various archaeal species, such as *Sulfolobus*, where conjugative plasmids like pNOB8 facilitate the exchange of DNA during cellular interaction [55, 56]. Research on *Sulfolobus acidocaldarius* has shown that conjugation can lead to extensive genomic recombination, enhancing genetic diversity within populations [55, 57]. Notably, studies of *E. coli* have shown its capacity to transfer DNA to a wide range of genetically distinct recipients, including archaea [58]. Additionally, studies have highlighted that conjugative mechanisms in archaea share similarities with bacterial conjugation systems, suggesting an evolutionary link between these processes [56, 59, 60].

Transformation is a fundamental mechanism for genetic exchange in prokaryotes. This process involves the uptake and integration of free DNA from the environment into a cell's genome, facilitating genetic diversity and adaptability. In archaea, transformation is often mediated by type IV pili, which play a crucial role in DNA transport and cell adhesion [59]. Research on the archaeon *Methanobacterium marburgensis* (formerly *Methanobacterium thermautotrophicum*), as well as *Methanosarcina mazei*, has demonstrated successful artificial transformation, highlighting the potential for genetic manipulation in these microorganisms [55, 61, 62]. Over the past 30 years, remarkable steps have been made in developing genetic systems for *Methanosarcina*. One major achievement is the establishment of DNA transformation methods [63] and markerless gene deletions have been successfully implemented [64–66]. Researchers have also generated shuttle vectors to enable efficient gene expression [67, 68]. More recently, genome editing using the Cas9 system has become possible [69]. Besides laboratory gene manipulation, some methanogenic archaea exhibit natural competence such as *M. marburgensis*, *Methanococcus voltae*. *Methanococcus maripaludis*, *Methanocellus thermophilus,* and *Thermococcus kodakarensis*, enabling efficient genetic modifications [70–72].

Beyond the well-known DNA transfer systems mentioned above, other mechanisms for DNA transfer have been identified in archaea. It is hypothesized that *Thermococcales* exchange plasmid DNA through the use of vesicles [73]. Further, the exchange of chromosomal DNA through spontaneous cell fusion processes was observed in *Haloarchaea* [74, 75]. Finally, members of *Sulfolobales* showed species-specific aggregates to exchange chromosomal DNA using proteins for DNA transport which was proposed as Crenarchaeal system for the exchange of DNA (Ced), although the precise mechanism is still not solved (**Figure 1**) [76].

2.3 Transposable elements in archaea

The mobility of genetic elements is not exclusively dependent on intercellular interactions of transposable elements in archaea, which act as important agents of genomic rearrangement and adaptation. The smallest representatives of TEs are miniature inverted-repeat transposable elements (MITEs) which are non-autonomous class II TEs. In case of MITEs, transposase genes are mutated up to partial or full deletions [1, 77]. In archaea, short insertion sequence (IS) elements represent the most abundant TEs showing similarities to bacterial IS-elements [1, 3], but their distribution is uneven across the archaeal domain, with a higher prevalence in orders such as *Halobacteriales*, *Sulfolobales*, *Thermoplasmatales*, and *Methanosarcinales* [3, 6–8]. Some archaeal genomes, like *M. marburgensis*, lack IS-elements entirely [1, 78, 79]. Deppenmeier and colleagues detected 102 transposases in the *M. mazei* genome [4]. S1-family transposons are one common group of TEs found in methanoarchaea e.g., *M. mazei*, *Methanosarcina barkeri*, and *Methanococcoides burtonii* [3]. Detection and quantification of TEs in archaea are biased due to the limited number of fully sequenced archaeal genomes and the tools used for prediction, likely leading to an underestimation of IS-element numbers and the representation of archaeal IS-element families [3, 32]. Unlike the well-studied eukaryotic TEs such as Tc1-mariner and Transib, archaeal TEs display unique structural and functional characteristics [3, 34, 80]. Classified by their catalytic motifs typical transposases which were detected in archaea belong to DDE transposases, serine (S) transposases and relaxase transposases [3]. The regulation of IS-element activity in archaea, while potentially linked to small non-coding RNAs (ncRNAs) regulating translation of transposase genes and translational readthrough, remains not fully understood. Observations in *M. barkeri* and *M. mazei* indicate that antisense RNAs (asRNAs) are primarily induced under stress conditions, implying that the regulation of IS elements through ncRNAs may be stress-dependent [3, 4, 81]. Additionally, during these stress responses, transposase activity tends to decrease, reducing the mobility of IS elements. This downregulation likely plays a role in preventing potential genomic instability, but the precise molecular mechanisms behind this remain to be clarified.

Early studies identified IS-elements in halophilic archaea, such as *Halobacterium salinarium* and *Halobacterium volcanii*, which harbor many MGEs causing significant genomic rearrangements [3, 82–86]. These elements were integrated into various chromosomal and plasmid sites, notably influencing phenotypes by disrupting operons like *gvp* and genes such as *bop* [87–92]. A link between high IS frequency and a challenging environment was observed in *Pyrococcus* isolates (36) from hydrothermal systems in the Pacific Ocean and the Mediterranean Sea (Vulcano Island). Using Multilocus sequence typing, it was found that *Pyrococcus* populations from different geographic locations were genetically distinct. The population from Vulcano Island had a notably high frequency of IS elements compared to populations in less challenging environments. This suggests that IS elements might play a role in driving genetic divergence between these geographically separated populations resulting in adaption [93]. Another example of evolving through genome plasticity like HGT and transposase activity is the psychrophile archaeon *M. burtonii* that potentially enable adaption to the cold as well as to biological and physical changes. To investigate the correlation between transposases and adaption, phylogenetic profiling was used to look for patterns of gene evolution. This demonstrated that transposases distinguish *M. burtonii* from other archaea, and their genomic characteristics indicate they have an important role in evolving the *M. burtonii* genome [94].

2.4 Casposons: A newly identified group of complex transposons in archaea

Casposons represent a fascinating class of TEs that bridge gaps between traditional transposons and the CRISPR-Cas adaptive immune systems in prokaryotes [95–105]. Discovered relatively recently, casposons stand out due to their exclusive structure and function, distinguishing them from other TEs. Recent studies have revealed that while most archaeal TEs show no significant similarity to eukaryotic elements, casposons share features with Polintons/Mavericks, including coding sequences for type B family DNA polymerases [35, 95, 106]. Besides, they are characterized by typical target site duplications (TSDs) and terminal inverted repeats (TIRs) similar to IS-elements but are unique in having multiple coding genes and a size extending to several kilobase pairs [95, 96]. These elements are primarily characterized by their encoding of a specific protein, Cas1 solo (or stand-alone Cas1) belonging to the Cas1-family, also referred to as casposase, which is essential for their transposition process. Classical Cas1 enzymes are essential components of the CRISPR-Cas immune system in prokaryotes, responsible for integrating new spacers into the CRISPR array during the adaptation phase of the immune response [101, 107]. Unlike classic transposons that encode conventional transposases, casposons lack these enzymes, highlighting their unique evolutionary pathway [95, 96, 98, 100, 108–110]. To date, four distinct casposon families have been identified, classified primarily by the domain structure of their Cas1 solo enzyme [96, 108].

The casposase enzyme encoded by casposons is thought to catalyze the excision and integration of these elements within the host genome. This process is hypothesized to be similar to the adaptation phase of the CRISPR-Cas immune response, where new spacers are integrated into the CRISPR array by Cas1-Cas2 [95–105]. The activity of Cas1 solo enzymes was postulated based on their conserved active site residues E141, H208, D218, and D221, homologous to those in CRISPR Cas1, and their presence in casposons supports an evolutionary link to CRISPR-Cas systems [95–97, 99–105, 108]. Consequently, casposons, in particular the casposon TIRs may have contributed to the development of CRISPR-Cas systems, potentially serving as a precursor or evolutionary ancestor to these adaptive immune systems [95–97, 99–101, 103–105, 108]. Krupovic and colleagues proposed a translocation model similar to the transposition of Polinton/Mavericks, predicting a TIR-mediated looping out of the casposon during cellular replication, followed by Cas1 solo-mediated excision, polB replication, and Cas1 solo-mediated reintegration into the genome [12, 95, 106, 111]. The reintegration, involving the generation of target site duplications, is proposed to function similarly to the spacer adaptation module of CRISPR systems [95]. Research involving heterologously expressed Cas1 solo enzymes has revealed their ability to excise and integrate casposon derivatives and small synthetic oligonucleotides *in vitro* [98, 100, 109, 110]. These studies primarily focus on analyzing Cas1 solo protein activities. Investigations into the casposon from the archeaon *Aciduliprofundum boonei*, particularly its Cas1 solo variant, have provided significant biochemical insights into the translocation mechanism and indicated possible *in vivo* activity [98, 100, 109]. Experiments with purified Cas1 solo from both *A. boonei* and *M. mazei* demonstrated that these enzymes can site-specifically integrate casposon derivatives or short synthetic oligonucleotides into various target sites on pUC19-derived plasmids *in vitro* [96, 98, 109, 110]. This site-specific integration process resembles the incorporation of new spacer sequences into CRISPR arrays during the CRISPR-Cas adaptation phase [95, 110]. Until recently, *in vivo* evidence for casposon activity has been lacking. In addition to the scarcity of suitable model systems and the limited number of genetically tractable hosts, a major challenge has been the absence of a selectable marker to detect casposon "hopping" or mobility. This limitation makes it difficult to directly observe integration events, assess their impact on growth or fitness, and detect potential loss of the casposon over time, as there is no clear selective advantage to track these changes [95, 96, 112]. Recently, the proposed *in vivo* translocation activity of the *M. mazei* casposon. MetMaz-C1 [96] was explored through a 472-day long-term evolution experiment (which corresponds to approximately 600 generations) [112]. MetMaz-C1 has a size of around 10 kb, encoding eight genes and is flanked by TIR of 31 nt and TSD of 14 nt [112]. The study with four different stress treatments (native conditions, high temperature, high salt, mitomycin C) examined and demonstrated translocation of the casposon employing an optimized nested qPCR to track casposon presence at various genomic sites and is now reported as an active MGE [112]. Moreover, in an independent approach the activity of a synthetic MetMaz-C1 derivative was tested using a mini-casposon assay, where the mini-casposon containing an R6Kγ origin and two antibiotic resistance genes flanked by TIRs and TSDs demonstrated active translocation from a suicide vector into the host genome [98, 100, 109, 110, 112]. Both methods confirmed precise casposon excision, leaving behind a single empty target site, and provided preliminary evidence for reintegration into new genomic loci, the formation of a possible circular intermediate, and the casposon's ability to create tandem structures by using the same target site repeatedly [112]. Furthermore, the long-term evolution experiment, using strains with and without Cas1solo overexpression, revealed differences in casposon excision frequencies under various stress conditions [112].

Casposons, with their distinct structural features and transposition mechanisms, provide valuable insights into the role of MGEs in genomic evolution. Their presence in archaea highlights the evolutionary relationships between MGEs and cellular processes, while also offering clues to the origins of complex gene-editing systems. Studies of casposons in mixed cultures could further enhance this aspect and future respective discoveries might deepen our understanding of casposons' influence on the genomic adaptability of archaea. Additionally, future studies should investigate the distribution and frequency of transposons in the currently available genomes to enable quantitative assessments.

2.5 Biotechnological applications of transposons

The development of genetic techniques for archaea has lagged behind the rapid advancements in molecular biology. As a result, we now encounter many instances where microbial genomes have been fully sequenced, but few or no genetic tools are available for those organisms. Transposons and casposons are valuable tools that have been widely used in bacteria, but their use in archaea has been much more limited. So far, only a few have been applied in archaea.

Using a modified mariner transposable element Himar1, originally found in the insect *Hematobia irritans* was implemented by Zhang et al. to allow *in vivo* transposon mutagenesis in the methanogenic archaeon *Methanosarcina acetivorans* C2A [113]. Modified mini-Himar1 elements were designed to include selectable markers functional in *Methanosarcina* species, along with the Himar1 transposase expressed from known *Methanosarcina* promoters. Due to its independence from host-specific factors, this system could potentially be widely applicable across various microorganisms [113]. Furthermore, the reprogrammed archaeal TnpB found on a short IS200/IS605 transposon in *Sulfolobus islandicus* REY15A is used for genome editing. It was taken advantage of that TnpB utilizes a single noncoding RNA to guide the cleavage of double-stranded DNA, demonstrating its genome editing capability in human cells [114].

Those are only some examples of how transposons are indispensable in many fields of research. Their ability to move within and between genomes has made them powerful tools for genetic studies, enabling scientists to investigate gene function, genome structure, and evolutionary processes. In biotechnology, transposons are used for mutagenesis, gene delivery, and genome editing. Moreover, their applications extend to medicine, where transposon-based systems are being developed.

3. Conclusions

In conclusion, the exploration of MGEs within archaea has revealed their profound influence on genetic diversity, adaptability, and evolution. MGEs, including plasmids, transposons, and casposons, play critical roles in shaping genomes, facilitating HGT, and driving the evolutionary processes that allow organisms to thrive in extreme environments. While much research has focused on bacterial and eukaryotic MGEs, recent studies on archaeal MGEs have highlighted their unique structural and functional characteristics, particularly in extremophiles. The classification and mechanisms of transposons show the complexity and diversity of these elements across different domains of life.

The discovery and analysis of casposons have provided new insights into the evolutionary link between transposons and the CRISPR-Cas adaptive immune systems, emphasizing the dynamic nature of genetic elements and their role in prokaryotic defense mechanisms.

As research continues to unravel the complexities of these elements, it is expected that new discoveries will deepen our knowledge of genome function and the intricate relationships between genetic elements and their hosts. MGEs, particularly in archaea, are poised to remain a crucial area of study, offering valuable insights into the mechanisms that drive genetic innovation and adaptation across all domains of life.

Conflict of interest

The authors declare no conflict of interest.

Author details

Luise Rentz, Finn O. Gehlert and Ruth A. Schmitz*
University of Kiel, Germany

*Address all correspondence to: rschmitz @ifam.uni-kiel.de

References

[1] Brügger K, Redder P, She Q, Confalonieri F, Zivanovic Y, Garrett RA. Mobile elements in archaeal genomes. FEMS Microbiology Letters. 2002;**206**:131-141

[2] Siguier P, Gourbeyre E, Varani A, Ton-Hoang B, Chandler M. Everyman's guide to bacterial insertion sequences. In: Craig NL, Chandler M, Gellert M, Lambowitz AM, Rice PA, Sandmeyer SB, editors. Mobile DNA III. Washington, DC, USA: ASM Press; 2015. pp. 555-590

[3] Filée J, Siguier P, Chandler M. Insertion sequence diversity in archaea. Microbiology and Molecular Biology Reviews MMBR. 2007;**71**:121-157

[4] Deppenmeier U, Johann A, Hartsch T, Merkl R, Schmitz RA, Martinez-Arias R, et al. The genome of *Methanosarcina mazei*: Evidence for lateral gene transfer between bacteria and archaea. Journal of Molecular Microbiology and Biotechnology. 2002;**4**:453-461

[5] Saralov AI. Adaptivity of archaeal and bacterial extremophiles. Microbiology. 2019;**88**:379-401

[6] Zhou F, Olman V, Xu Y. Insertion sequences show diverse recent activities in cyanobacteria and archaea. BMC Genomics. 2008;**9**:36

[7] She Q, Singh RK, Confalonieri F, Zivanovic Y, Allard G, Awayez MJ, et al. The complete genome of the crenarchaeon *Sulfolobus solfataricus* P2. Proceedings of the National Academy of Sciences of the United States of America. 2001;**98**:7835-7840

[8] Ng WV, Kennedy SP, Mahairas GG, Berquist B, Pan M, Shukla HD, et al. Genome sequence of *Halobacterium* species NRC-1. Proceedings of the National Academy of Sciences of the United States of America. 2000;**97**:12176-12181

[9] Hüttermann J. Methanoarchaeal Gene Expression: Innovations and Improvements for Biotechnological Application [Doctoral thesis]. Kiel: Johanna Hüttermann; 2024 [unpublished]

[10] Couturier M, Bex F, Bergquist PL, Maas WK. Identification and classification of bacterial plasmids. Microbiological Reviews. 1988;**52**:375-395

[11] Hinnebusch J, Tilly K. Linear plasmids and chromosomes in bacteria. Molecular Microbiology. 1993;**10**:917-922

[12] Meinhardt F, Kempken F, Kämper J, Esser K. Linear plasmids among eukaryotes: Fundamentals and application. Current Genetics. 1990;**17**:89-95

[13] Sakaguchi K. Invertrons, a class of structurally and functionally related genetic elements that includes linear DNA plasmids, transposable elements, and genomes of adeno-type viruses. Microbiological Reviews. 1990;**54**:66-74

[14] Frost LS, Leplae R, Summers AO, Toussaint A. Mobile genetic elements: The agents of open source evolution. Nature Reviews. Microbiology. 2005;**3**:722-732

[15] Arnold HP, She Q, Phan H, Stedman K, Prangishvili D, Holz I, et al. The genetic element pSSVx of the extremely thermophilic crenarchaeon Sulfolobus is a hybrid between a plasmid and a virus. Molecular Microbiology. 1999;**34**:217-226

[16] Zillig W, Kletzin A, Schleper C, Holz I, Janekovic D, Hain J, et al. Screening for sulfolobales, their plasmids and their viruses in Icelandic Solfataras. Systematic and Applied Microbiology. 1993;**16**:609-628

[17] Greve B, Jensen S, Phan H, Brügger K, Zillig W, She Q, et al. Novel RepA-MCM proteins encoded in plasmids pTAU4, pORA1 and pTIK4 from *Sulfolobus neozealandicus*. Archaea (Vancouver, B.C.). 2005;**1**:319-325

[18] McCLINTOCK B. The origin and behavior of mutable loci in maize. Proceedings of the National Academy of Sciences of the United States of America. 1950;**36**:344-355

[19] McClintock B. Controlling elements and the gene. Cold Spring Harbor Symposia on Quantitative Biology. 1956;**21**:197-216

[20] McClintock B. The significance of responses of the genome to challenge. Science (New York, N.Y.). 1984;**226**:792-801

[21] Huda A, Jordan IK. Epigenetic regulation of mammalian genomes by transposable elements. Annals of the New York Academy of Sciences. 2009;**1178**:276-284

[22] Schnable PS, Ware D, Fulton RS, Stein JC, Wei F, Pasternak S, et al. The B73 maize genome: Complexity, diversity, and dynamics. Science (New York, N.Y.). 2009;**326**:1112-1115

[23] Grabundzija I, Messing SA, Thomas J, Cosby RL, Bilic I, Miskey C, et al. A Helitron transposon reconstructed from bats reveals a novel mechanism of genome shuffling in eukaryotes. Nature Communications. 2016;**7**:10716

[24] Higgins BP, Carpenter CD, Karls AC. Chromosomal context directs high-frequency precise excision of IS492 in *Pseudoalteromonas atlantica*. Proceedings of the National Academy of Sciences of the United States of America. 2007;**104**:1901-1906

[25] Perkins-Balding D, Duval-Valentin G, Glasgow AC. Excision of IS492 requires flanking target sequences and results in circle formation in *Pseudoalteromonas atlantica*. Journal of Bacteriology. 1999;**181**:4937-4948

[26] Horne T, Orr VT, Hall JPJ. How do interactions between mobile genetic elements affect horizontal gene transfer? Current Opinion in Microbiology. 2023;**73**:102282

[27] Wicker T, Sabot F, Hua-Van A, Bennetzen JL, Capy P, Chalhoub B, et al. A unified classification system for eukaryotic transposable elements. Nature Reviews. Genetics. 2007;**8**:973-982

[28] Finnegan DJ. Eukaryotic transposable elements and genome evolution, trends in genetics. TIG. 1989;**5**:103-107

[29] Krupovic M, Bamford DH, Koonin EV. Conservation of major and minor jelly-roll capsid proteins in Polinton (maverick) transposons suggests that they are bona fide viruses. Biology Direct. 2014;**9**:6

[30] Luschnig C, Bachmair A. RNA packaging of yeast retrotransposon Ty1 in the heterologous host, *Escherichia coli*. Biological Chemistry. 1997;**378**:39-46

[31] Kapitonov VV, Jurka J. A universal classification of eukaryotic transposable elements implemented in Repbase, nature reviews. Genetics. 2008;**9**:411-412. author reply 414

[32] Arkhipova IR. Using bioinformatic and phylogenetic approaches to classify

transposable elements and understand their complex evolutionary histories. Mobile DNA. 2017;**8**:19

[33] Boeke JD, Garfinkel DJ, Styles CA, Fink GR. Ty elements transpose through an RNA intermediate. Cell. 1985;**40**:491-500

[34] Shao H, Tu Z. Expanding the diversity of the IS630-Tc1-mariner superfamily: Discovery of a unique DD37E transposon and reclassification of the DD37D and DD39D transposons. Genetics. 2001;**159**:1103-1115

[35] Pritham EJ, Putliwala T, Feschotte C. Mavericks, a novel class of giant transposable elements widespread in eukaryotes and related to DNA viruses. Gene. 2007;**390**:3-17

[36] Bennetzen JL. The contributions of retroelements to plant genome organization, function and evolution. Trends in Microbiology. 1996;**4**:347-353

[37] SanMiguel P. Evidence that a recent increase in maize genome size was caused by the massive amplification of intergene retrotransposons. Annals of Botany. 1998;**82**:37-44

[38] Bennetzen JL, Hake S. Handbook of Maize: History and Practice of Genetics and Genomics. New York: Springer; 2009

[39] Meyers BC, Tingey SV, Morgante M. Abundance, distribution, and transcriptional activity of repetitive elements in the maize genome. Genome Research. 2001;**11**:1660-1676

[40] Adams MD, Celniker SE, Holt RA, Evans CA, Gocayne JD, Amanatides PG, et al. The genome sequence of *Drosophila melanogaster*. Science (New York, N.Y.). 2000;**287**:2185-2195

[41] Bourque G, Burns KH, Gehring M, Gorbunova V, Seluanov A, Hammell M, et al. Ten things you should know about transposable elements. Genome Biology. 2018;**19**:199

[42] Canchaya C, Fournous G, Chibani-Chennoufi S, Dillmann ML, Brüssow H. Phage as agents of lateral gene transfer. Current Opinion in Microbiology. 2003;**6**:417-424

[43] Hodgson DA. Generalized transduction of serotype 1/2 and serotype 4b strains of *Listeria monocytogenes*. Molecular Microbiology. 2000;**35**:312-323

[44] Burke J, Schneider D, Westpheling J. Generalized transduction in *Streptomyces coelicolor*. Proceedings of the National Academy of Sciences of the United States of America. 2001;**98**:6289-6294

[45] Sander M, Schmieger H. Method for host-independent detection of generalized transducing bacteriophages in natural habitats. Applied and Environmental Microbiology. 2001;**67**:1490-1493

[46] Echols H, Green L. Establishment and maintenance of repression by bacteriophage lambda: The role of the cI, cII, and c3 proteins. Proceedings of the National Academy of Sciences of the United States of America. 1971;**68**:2190-2194

[47] Erez Z, Steinberger-Levy I, Shamir M, Doron S, Stokar-Avihail A, Peleg Y, et al. Communication between viruses guides lysis-lysogeny decisions. Nature. 2017;**541**:488-493

[48] Silpe JE, Bassler BL. A host-produced quorum-sensing autoinducer controls a phage lysis-lysogeny decision. Cell. 2019;**176**:268-280.e13

[49] Krupovic M, Cvirkaite-Krupovic V, Iranzo J, Prangishvili D, Koonin EV.

Viruses of archaea: Structural, functional, environmental and evolutionary genomics. Virus Research. 2018;**244**:181-193

[50] Dellas N, Snyder JC, Bolduc B, Young MJ. Archaeal viruses: Diversity. Replication, and Structure, Annual review of virology. 2014;**1**:399-426

[51] Torsvik T, Dundas ID. Bacteriophage of *Halobacterium salinarium*. Nature. 1974;**248**:680-681

[52] Held NL, Herrera A, Cadillo-Quiroz H, Whitaker RJ. CRISPR associated diversity within a population of *Sulfolobus islandicus*. PLoS One. 2010;**5**:e12988

[53] Krupovic M, Prangishvili D, Hendrix RW, Bamford DH. Genomics of bacterial and archaeal viruses: Dynamics within the prokaryotic virosphere. Microbiology and Molecular Biology Reviews MMBR. 2011;**75**:610-635

[54] Prangishvili D, Forterre P, Garrett RA. Viruses of the archaea: A unifying view. Nature Reviews. Microbiology. 2006;**4**:837-848

[55] Leigh JA, Albers S-V, Atomi H, Allers T. Model organisms for genetics in the domain archaea: Methanogens, halophiles, *Thermococcales* and *Sulfolobales*. FEMS Microbiology Reviews. 2011;**35**:577-608

[56] Averhoff B, Friedrich A. Type IV pili-related natural transformation systems: DNA transport in mesophilic and thermophilic bacteria. Archives of Microbiology. 2003;**180**:385-393

[57] Hansen JE, Dill AC, Grogan DW. Conjugational genetic exchange in the hyperthermophilic archaeon *Sulfolobus acidocaldarius*: Intragenic recombination with minimal dependence on marker separation. Journal of Bacteriology. 2005;**187**:805-809

[58] Dodsworth JA, Li L, Wei S, Hedlund BP, Leigh JA, de Figueiredo P. Interdomain conjugal transfer of DNA from bacteria to archaea. Applied and Environmental Microbiology. 2010;**76**:5644-5647

[59] Wagner A, Whitaker RJ, Krause DJ, Heilers J-H, van Wolferen M, van der Does C, et al. Mechanisms of gene flow in archaea. Nature Reviews. Microbiology. 2017;**15**:492-501

[60] Peng N, Han W, Li Y, Liang Y, She Q. Genetic technologies for extremely thermophilic microorganisms of Sulfolobus, the only genetically tractable genus of crenarchaea, science China. Life Sciences. 2017;**60**:370-385

[61] Contreras G, Thomsen J, Pfitzer M, Hafenbradl D, Kostner D, Holtmann D, et al. New perspectives for biotechnological applications of methanogens. Current Research in Biotechnology. 2022;**4**:468-474

[62] Kohler PRA, Metcalf WW. Genetic manipulation of *Methanosarcina* spp. Frontiers in Microbiology. 2012;**3**:259

[63] Ehlers C, Weidenbach K, Veit K, Deppenmeier U, Metcalf WW, Schmitz RA. Development of genetic methods and construction of a chromosomal glnK1 mutant in *Methanosarcina mazei* strain Gö1, molecular genetics and genomics. MGG. 2005;**273**:290-298

[64] Ehlers C, Jäger D, Schmitz RA. Establishing a markerless genetic exchange system for *Methanosarcina mazei* strain Gö1 for constructing chromosomal mutants of small RNA genes. Archaea (Vancouver, B.C.). 2011;**2011**:439608

[65] Pritchett MA, Zhang JK, Metcalf WW. Development of a markerless genetic exchange method for *Methanosarcina acetivorans* C2A and its use in construction of new genetic tools for methanogenic archaea. Applied and Environmental Microbiology. 2004;**70**:1425-1433

[66] Thomsen J, Weidenbach K, Metcalf WW, Schmitz RA. Genetic methods and construction of chromosomal mutations in methanogenic archaea. Methods in Molecular Biology (Clifton, N.J.). 2022;**2522**:105-117

[67] Metcalf WW, Zhang JK, Apolinario E, Sowers KR, Wolfe RS. A genetic system for archaea of the genus Methanosarcina: Liposome-mediated transformation and construction of shuttle vectors. Proceedings of the National Academy of Sciences of the United States of America. 1997;**94**:2626-2631

[68] Thomsen J, Schmitz RA. Generating a small shuttle vector for effective genetic engineering of *Methanosarcina mazei* allowed first insights in plasmid replication mechanism in the Methanoarchaeon. International Journal of Molecular Sciences. 2022;**23**:2-4

[69] Nayak DD, Metcalf WW. Cas9-mediated genome editing in the methanogenic archaeon *Methanosarcina acetivorans*. Proceedings of the National Academy of Sciences of the United States of America. 2017;**114**:2976-2981

[70] Fonseca DR, Halim MFA, Holten MP, Costa KC. Type IV-like pili facilitate transformation in naturally competent archaea. Journal of Bacteriology. 2020;**202**:2-9

[71] Hileman TH, Santangelo TJ. Genetics techniques for *Thermococcus kodakarensis*. Frontiers in Microbiology. 2012;**3**:195

[72] Gophna U, Altman-Price N. Horizontal gene transfer in archaea-from mechanisms to genome evolution. Annual Review of Microbiology. 2022;**76**:481-502

[73] Gaudin M, Gauliard E, Schouten S, Houel-Renault L, Lenormand P, Marguet E, et al. Hyperthermophilic archaea produce membrane vesicles that can transfer DNA. Environmental Microbiology Reports. 2013;**5**:109-116

[74] Naor A, Lapierre P, Mevarech M, Papke RT, Gophna U. Low species barriers in halophilic archaea and the formation of recombinant hybrids. Current Biology CB. 2012;**22**:1444-1448

[75] Naor A, Gophna U. Cell fusion and hybrids in archaea: Prospects for genome shuffling and accelerated strain development for biotechnology. Bioengineered. 2013;**4**:126-129

[76] van Wolferen M, Wagner A, van der Does C, Albers S-V. The archaeal Ced system imports DNA. Proceedings of the National Academy of Sciences of the United States of America. 2016;**113**:2496-2501

[77] Redder P, She Q, Garrett RA. Non-autonomous mobile elements in the crenarchaeon *Sulfolobus solfataricus*. Journal of Molecular Biology. 2001;**306**:1-6

[78] Smith DR, Doucette-Stamm LA, Deloughery C, Lee H, Dubois J, Aldredge T, et al. Complete genome sequence of *Methanobacterium* thermoautotrophicum deltaH: Functional analysis and comparative genomics. Journal of Bacteriology. 1997;**179**:7135-7155

[79] Liesegang H, Kaster A-K, Wiezer A, Goenrich M, Wollherr A, Seedorf H, et al. Complete genome

sequence of *Methanothermobacter marburgensis*, a methanoarchaeon model organism. Journal of Bacteriology. 2010;**192**:5850-5851

[80] Pritham EJ, Feschotte C, Wessler SR. Unexpected diversity and differential success of DNA transposons in four species of entamoeba protozoans. Molecular Biology and Evolution. 2005;**22**:1751-1763

[81] Jäger D, Sharma CM, Thomsen J, Ehlers C, Vogel J, Schmitz RA. Deep sequencing analysis of the *Methanosarcina mazei* Gö1 transcriptome in response to nitrogen availability. Proceedings of the National Academy of Sciences of the United States of America. 2009;**106**:21878-21882

[82] Ng WV, Ciufo SA, Smith TM, Bumgarner RE, Baskin D, Faust J, et al. Snapshot of a large dynamic replicon in a halophilic archaeon: Megaplasmid or minichromosome? Genome Research. 1998;**8**:1131-1141

[83] Pfeifer F, Weidinger G, Goebel W. Characterization of plasmids in halobacteria. Journal of Bacteriology. 1981;**145**:369-374

[84] Pfeifer F, Weidinger G, Goebel W. Genetic variability in *Halobacterium halobium*. Journal of Bacteriology. 1981;**145**:375-381

[85] Pfeifer F, Blaseio U. Transposition burst of the ISH27 insertion element family in *Halobacterium halobium*. Nucleic Acids Research. 1990;**18**:6921-6925

[86] Sapienza C, Rose MR, Doolittle WF. High-frequency genomic rearrangements involving archaebacterial repeat sequence elements. Nature. 1982;**299**:182-185

[87] Halladay JT, Jones JG, Lin F, MacDonald AB, DasSarma S. The rightward gas vesicle operon in *Halobacterium* plasmid pNRC100: Identification of the gvpA and gvpC gene products by use of antibody probes and genetic analysis of the region downstream of gvpC. Journal of Bacteriology. 1993;**175**:684-692

[88] DasSarma S, RajBhandary UL, Khorana HG. High-frequency spontaneous mutation in the bacterio-opsin gene in *Halobacterium halobium* is mediated by transposable elements. Proceedings of the National Academy of Sciences of the United States of America. 1983;**80**:2201-2205

[89] Pfeifer F, Friedman J, Boyer HW, Betlach M. Characterization of insertions affecting the expression of the bacterio-opsin gene in *Halobacterium halobium*. Nucleic Acids Research. 1984;**12**:2489-2497

[90] Krebs MP, RajBhandary UL, Khorana HG. Nucleotide sequence of ISH11, a new *Halobacterium halobium* insertion element isolated from the plasmid pGRB1. Nucleic Acids Research. 1990;**18**:6699

[91] DasSarma S. Mechanisms of genetic variability in *Halobacterium halobium*: The purple membrane and gas vesicle mutations. Canadian Journal of Microbiology. 1989;**35**:65-72

[92] Pfeifer F, Blaseio U, Ghahraman P. Dynamic plasmid populations in *Halobacterium halobium*. Journal of Bacteriology. 1988;**170**:3718-3724

[93] Escobar-Páramo P, Ghosh S, DiRuggiero J. Evidence for genetic drift in the diversification of a geographically isolated population of the hyperthermophilic archaeon *Pyrococcus*. Molecular Biology and Evolution. 2005;**22**:2297-2303

[94] Allen MA, Lauro FM, Williams TJ, Burg D, Siddiqui KS, de Francisci D, et al. The genome sequence of the psychrophilic archaeon, *Methanococcoides burtonii*: The role of genome evolution in cold adaptation. The ISME Journal. 2009;**3**:1012-1035

[95] Krupovic M, Makarova KS, Forterre P, Prangishvili D, Koonin EV. Casposons: A new superfamily of self-synthesizing DNA transposons at the origin of prokaryotic CRISPR-Cas immunity. BMC Biology. 2014;**12**:36

[96] Krupovic M, Shmakov S, Makarova KS, Forterre P, Koonin EV. Recent mobility of Casposons, self-synthesizing transposons at the origin of the CRISPR-Cas immunity. Genome Biology and Evolution. 2016;**8**:375-386

[97] Krupovic M, Koonin EV. Self-synthesizing transposons: Unexpected key players in the evolution of viruses and defense systems. Current Opinion in Microbiology. 2016;**31**:25-33

[98] Béguin P, Charpin N, Koonin EV, Forterre P, Krupovic M. Casposon integration shows strong target site preference and recapitulates protospacer integration by CRISPR-Cas systems. Nucleic Acids Research. 2016;**44**:10367-10376

[99] Hickman AB, Dyda F. CRISPR-Cas immunity and mobile DNA: A new superfamily of DNA transposons encoding a Cas1 endonuclease. Mobile DNA. 2014;**5**:23

[100] Hickman AB, Dyda F. The casposon-encoded Cas1 protein from *Aciduliprofundum boonei* is a DNA integrase that generates target site duplications. Nucleic Acids Research. 2015;**43**:10576-10587

[101] Makarova KS, Wolf YI, Koonin EV. The basic building blocks and evolution of CRISPR-CAS systems. Biochemical Society Transactions. 2013;**41**:1392-1400

[102] Babu M, Beloglazova N, Flick R, Graham C, Skarina T, Nocek B, et al. A dual function of the CRISPR-Cas system in bacterial antivirus immunity and DNA repair. Molecular Microbiology. 2011;**79**:484-502

[103] Nuñez JK, Kranzusch PJ, Noeske J, Wright AV, Davies CW, Doudna JA. Cas1-Cas2 complex formation mediates spacer acquisition during CRISPR-Cas adaptive immunity. Nature Structural & Molecular Biology. 2014;**21**:528-534

[104] Nuñez JK, Lee ASY, Engelman A, Doudna JA. Integrase-mediated spacer acquisition during CRISPR-Cas adaptive immunity. Nature. 2015;**519**:193-198

[105] Rollie C, Schneider S, Brinkmann AS, Bolt EL, White MF. Intrinsic sequence specificity of the Cas1 integrase directs new spacer acquisition. eLife. 2015;**4**:e08716

[106] Kapitonov VV, Jurka J. Self-synthesizing DNA transposons in eukaryotes. Proceedings of the National Academy of Sciences of the United States of America. 2006;**103**:4540-4545

[107] Makarova KS, Aravind L, Wolf YI, Koonin EV. Unification of Cas protein families and a simple scenario for the origin and evolution of CRISPR-Cas systems. Biology Direct. 2011;**6**:38

[108] Krupovic M, Béguin P, Koonin EV. Casposons: Mobile genetic elements that gave rise to the CRISPR-Cas adaptation machinery. Current Opinion in Microbiology. 2017;**38**:36-43

[109] Béguin P, Chekli Y, Sezonov G, Forterre P, Krupovic M. Sequence motifs recognized by the casposon integrase of *Aciduliprofundum boonei*. Nucleic Acids Research. 2019;**47**:6386-6395

[110] Hickman AB, Kailasan S, Genzor P, Haase AD, Dyda F. Casposase structure and the mechanistic link between DNA transposition and spacer acquisition by CRISPR-Cas. eLife. 2020;**9**:3-19

[111] Salas M. Protein-priming of DNA replication. Annual Review of Biochemistry. 1991;**60**:39-71

[112] Gehlert FO, Nickel L, Vakirlis N, Hammerschmidt K, Vargas Gebauer HI, Kießling C, et al. Active in vivo translocation of the *Methanosarcina mazei* Gö1 Casposon. Nucleic Acids Research. 2023;**51**:6927-6943

[113] Zhang JK, Pritchett MA, Lampe DJ, Robertson HM, Metcalf WW. In vivo transposon mutagenesis of the methanogenic archaeon *Methanosarcina acetivorans* C2A using a modified version of the insect mariner -family transposable element Himar1. Proceedings. National Academy of Sciences. United States of America. 2000;**97**:9665-9670

[114] Xu Y, Liu T, Wang J, Xiong B, Liu L, Peng N. Reprogramming an RNA-guided archaeal TnpB endonuclease for genome editing. Cell Discovery. 2023;**9**:112

Chapter 4

Co-Production of Hydrogen and Methane by Anaerobic Digestion

Fang Yin, Junlin Ji and Wudi Zhang

Abstract

According to the analysis of material metabolic pathway, mutual symbiotic flora, and energy cooperative sharing, the paper proposed that the ideal anaerobic digestion metabolism process of hydrogen production followed by methane production coincided with the mutual symbiotic and synergistic mechanism. (1) Hydrogen, carbon dioxide, and acetate acid are the important intermediates in the process of anaerobic digestion for co-production of methane and hydrogen. (2) Hydrogen-producing acetogenic, bacteria and hydrogen-consuming methanogenic bacteria undergo mutual coupling to become the anaerobic symbiotic compact, sharing organic material degradation and contributing chemical energy (15 kJ/mol). (3) From the point of view of adenosine triphosphate (ATP) energetics, we explain the phenomenon of low energy dissipations of anaerobic digestion, which is about 20 kJ/mol of energy requirements for symbiotic community survival. The viewpoint of mutual symbiosis was supported by the typical case of mutual symbiotic community in the 1960s and H_2 hypothesis in the 1970s' which also verified the optimal energy conversion efficiency of co-production of hydrogen and methane.

Keywords: anaerobic metabolism, co-production of hydrogen and methane, cooperative energy sharing, symbiotic microbial, mutualism

1. Introduction

1.1 Significate of co-production of hydrogen and methane by methanogenic metabolism

In the early 1990s, the production of biological hydrogen by fermentation of organic wastewater drew attention [1]. The physiological and ecological theory of acidogenic fermentation of microorganisms was presented, and a series of hydrogen-producing technologies of biological fermentation were implemented by exploiting the acidogenic fermentation effect of acidogenic bacteria. In their proposition regarding the hydrogen production efficiency of the biological fermentation hydrogen production system to address the key technical issues, the hydrogen conversion efficiency per unit substrate (measured in glucose G) is extremely low, merely 2 mol/molG, and the majority of the hydrogen in the raw material is still fixed in the fermentation products, such as propionic acid, butyric acid, lactic acid, and ethanol. There are microflora with complex population relationships within the fermentation system. Hydrogen-producing acetogenic bacteria are capable of converting propionic acid, butyric acid, and ethanol into acetic acid, hydrogen (H_2), and carbon dioxide (CO_2). With the assistance of the stepwise degradation of glucose by fermentation of acidogenic bacteria and hydrogen-producing acidogenic bacteria, the hydrogen conversion rate of the substrate can reach over 2.5 mol/molG. How to break through the metabolic barrier of anaerobic activated sludge to biomass fermentation hydrogen production and enhance the hydrogen conversion rate per unit substrate has emerged as the bottleneck restricting the hydrogen-producing technologies of biological fermentation [2].

Utilizing *Eupatorium adenophorum* Spreng. as the feedstock, the raw materials (cellulose, hemicellulose, and lignin) were analyzed and assessed through a sequential fermentation process of hydrogen production followed by methane production, as well as methane production followed by hydrogen production. Concurrently, gas generation and gas production rate were evaluated and compared. It was observed that adopting the pathway of hydrogen production followed by methane production enhanced the degradation efficiency of raw materials within the fermentation system, thus representing a rational material flow route.

2. Energy efficiency analysis of joint production of hydrogen and methane

By comparing and analyzing the productivity efficiency of fermentation systems, it was determined that the anaerobic digestion degradation mode involving hydrogen production prior to methane production exhibits an optimal and efficient performance [3]. This mode demonstrates a rational metabolic flow path for anaerobic digestion compared to the alternative approach of hydrogen production after methane production, thereby aligning with the energy sharing mechanism.

2.1 Potential for producing hydrogen and methane

In Experiment 1, hydrogen fermentation was conducted first. After hydrogen production ended, the pH was adjusted to 7 and then methane fermentation was carried out. The experiment was conducted for a total of 50 days (**Figure 1**).

In Experiment 2, methane fermentation was conducted first. After methane production ended, the pH was adjusted to 5 and then hydrogen fermentation was carried out. The experiment was conducted for a total of 669 days (**Figure 2**).

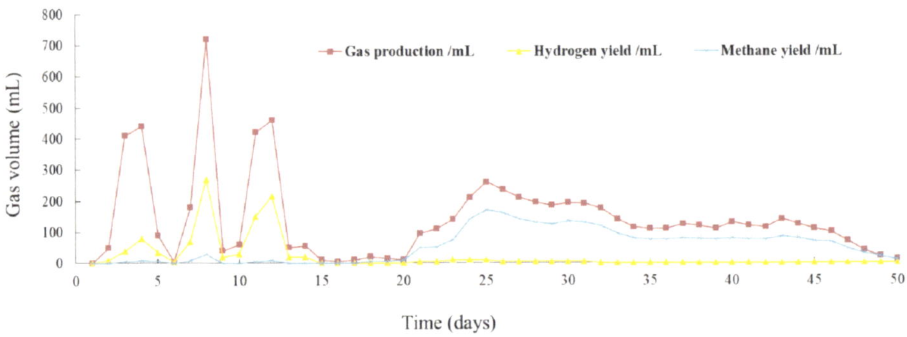

Figure 1.
Gas production curve in Experiment 1.

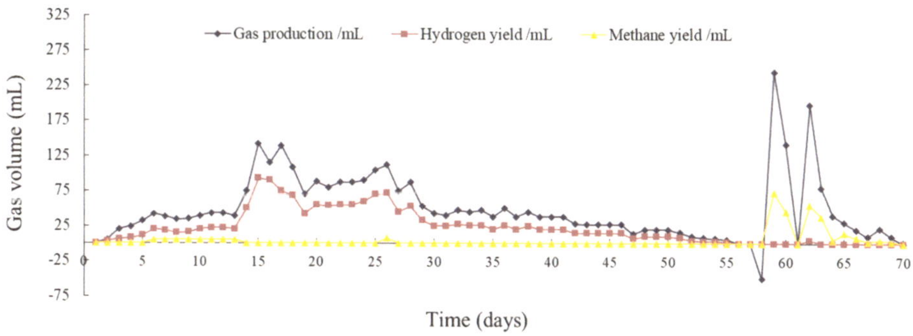

Figure 2.
Gas production curve in Experiment 2.

The gas production rates of total solids (TS) and volatile solids (VS) in each stage of Experiment 1 are observed to be higher than those of Experiment 2, as indicated by the data presented in **Table 1**.

2.2 Comparative analysis of raw material utilization

The contents of cellulose, hemicellulose, and lignin in fermentation raw materials, inoculants, and feed liquid before and after fermentation were determined, as shown in **Table 2**.

The utilization rate of raw materials (cellulose, hemicellulose, and lignin) in each stage of Experiment 1 is observed to be higher than that in Experiment 2, as indicated by the data presented in **Table 2**.

2.3 Characteristics of hydrogen production stage

Hydrogen-producing acetogenic bacteria and methanogenic bacteria are interdependent and mutually constrained in a fermentation system, and the "interspecies hydrogen transfer" between them allows the hydrogen-producing bacteria to continuously provide hydrogen, while the methanogenic bacteria continuously consume hydrogen. By artificially regulating the pH of the system, a dynamic balance between hydrogen production and utilization can be achieved [4].

Adjust the pH of the fermentation system with acetic acid (HAc) and hydrochloric acid (HCl), respectively. Compared with the HCl regulation method, the fermentation with HAc-adjusted pH had a better gas production effect, while the fermentation with HCl-adjusted pH started faster. The cellulose degradation rate regulated by HAc is higher than that regulated by HCl, and the energy conversion and utilization effect of the system is better.

2.3.1 Terminal judgment of hydrogen production stage

The gas production during the hydrogen production stage in Experiment 1 and Experiment 2 is shown in **Figures 3** and **4**. It can be seen from the figures that there is a peak in gas production every time the pH is adjusted. The gas production of the experimental group is higher than that of the control group, but the difference in gas production between the experimental group and the control group is significantly reduced in the later stage. The peak of gas production in the experimental group

Test		Total gas production/mL	H_2 content /%	CH_4 content /%	Daily gas production/mL	TS gas production rate/L kg^{-1}	VS gas production rate/L kg^{-1}	Daily gas production rate/ mL mL^{-1} d^{-1}
Experiment 1	Hydrogen production stage	3010	30.85	2.31	215	49.09	63.66	0.13
	Methane production stage	4143	2.38	61.74	115.09	135.21	175.35	0.14
Experiment 2	Methane production stage	2744	1.18	62.44	49.01	101.91	127.82	0.061
	Hydrogen production stage	738	32.26	1.63	56.79	14.16	17.77	0.037

Table 1.
Potential for producing hydrogen and methane of Eupatorium adenophorum *Sprend by anaerobic digestion.*

Measurement indicators		Cellulose content (%)	Hemicellulose content (%)	Lignin content (%)
Experiment 1	Raw material	30.08	22.43	21.99
	Before/after hydrogen production fermentation	28.09/26.72	19.88/17.52	20.76/20.33
	Utilization rate of hydrogen production stage	4.88	11.87	2.07
	Before/after methane fermentation	26.72/22.48	17.52/14.57	20.33/18.96
	Utilization rate of methane production stage	15.87	16.84	6.74
Experiment 2	Raw material	31.42	24.61	20.93
	Before/after methane fermentation	26.96/23.21	20.48/16.96	19.41/18.41
	Utilization rate of methane production stage	13.83	16.66	5.41
	Before/after hydrogen production fermentation	23.21/22.88	16.96/16.52	18.41/18.34
	Utilization rate of hydrogen production stage	1.42	2.59	0.38

Table 2.
Analysis of cellulose, hemicellulose, and lignin content.

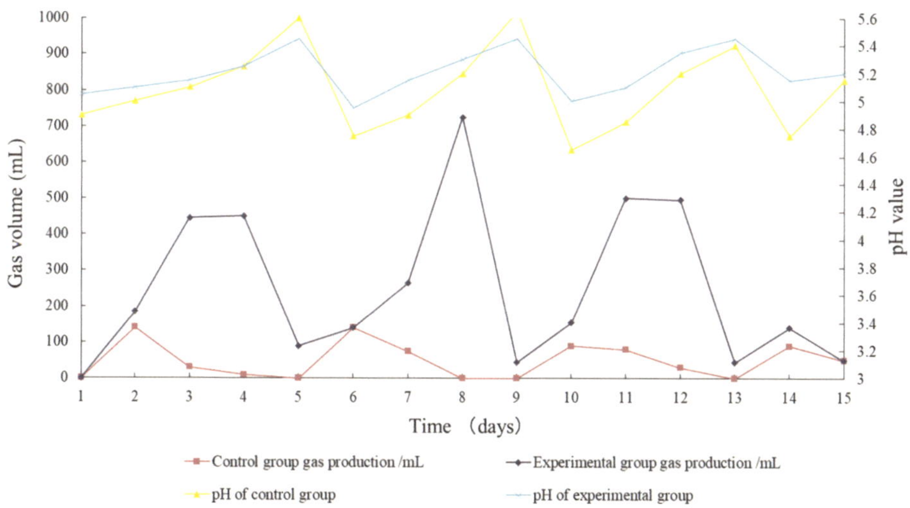

Figure 3.
Gas production curve of hydrogen production stage in Experiment 1.

occurred after the peak of gas production in the control group, and the increase of pH in the control group was higher than that in the experimental group, which may be due to the microbial community in the control group being in a nutrient-deficient environment, and the lactic acid used to regulate pH could be used as a carbon source

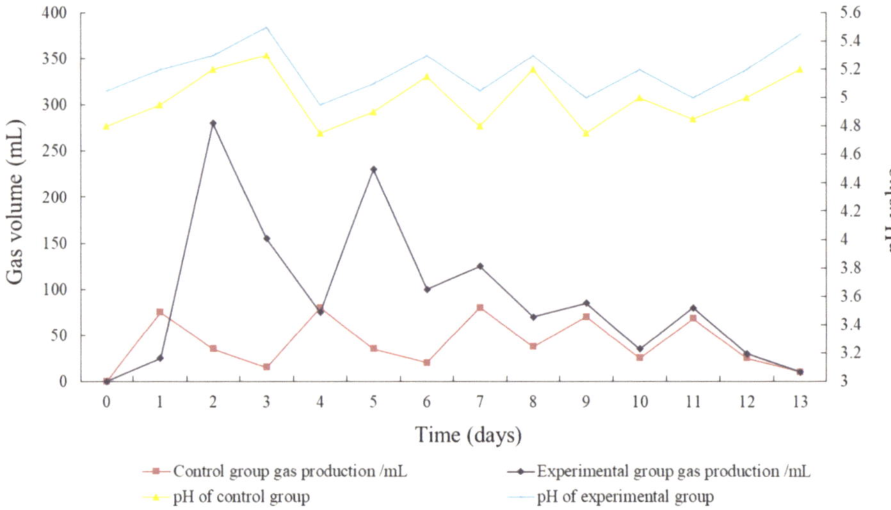

Figure 4.
Gas production curve of hydrogen production stage in Experiment 2.

for its metabolism. In the environment where the microbial community of the experimental group is located, the substances that are more easily decomposed in the raw materials can become their metabolic raw materials, and the rate of consumption of lactic acid is lower than that of the control group, resulting in a slower increase in the pH of the system.

It can be determined whether the hydrogen production stage is complete by assessing whether the gas production trends of the experimental and control groups align. As shown in **Figure 4**, on the seventh day, when the gas production trends of both groups converged, further lactic acid additions were made to adjust pH and extend the fermentation period. The gas production trends of both groups continued to converge, with the experimental group no longer showing a significant production advantage over the control group, indicating that fermentation had been completed.

2.3.2 Comparison of raw material utilization in hydrogen production stage

There is a difference between the hydrogen production effect of direct fermentation and the hydrogen production after methane fermentation. Assuming the index values in the hydrogen production stage of Experiment 1 are 1, we can visually compare the differences between the two processes by referring to Experiment 1's index values, as illustrated in **Figure 5**.

If hydrogen is first produced through fermentation, the acidic environment of the system is conducive to the accumulation of hydrogen-producing bacteria and intermediate metabolites, especially acetic acid and butyric acid, which determine the amount of hydrogen produced. If methane is first produced through fermentation, the metabolites in the system, including ethanol, acetic acid, pyruvic acid, butyric acid, and other organic acids, are initially converted into methane, and then the pH value is adjusted to produce hydrogen. The acidic environment restimulates the accumulation of hydrogen-producing bacteria and hydrogen-producing intermediate metabolites in the system, so that the remaining organic acids can be finally converted into hydrogen.

The utilization rate of raw materials for hydrogen production through initial fermentation is observed to be higher than that for biogas production followed by

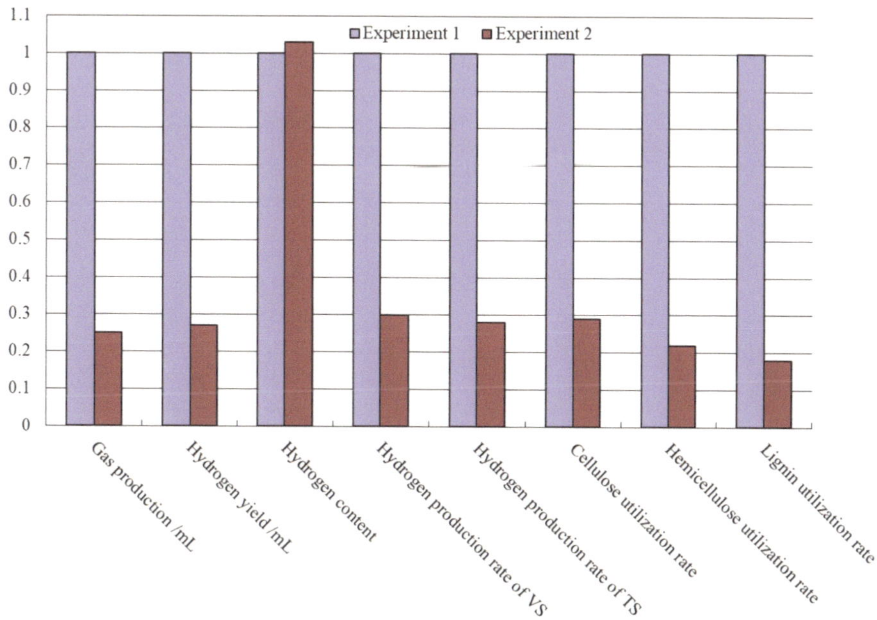

Figure 5.
Comparison of various indicators during hydrogen production.

hydrogen generation, as depicted in **Figure 5**. The acidic environment during the hydrogen production stage facilitates the degradation and utilization of raw materials, such as cellulose, hemicellulose, and lignin.

2.4 Characteristics of methane production stage

2.4.1 Comparison of raw material utilization in methane production stage

The methanogenic effects differ between the two processes: fermentation of first producing hydrogen then methane and fermentation of directly producing methane from raw materials. Taking the index values in the methane production stage of Experiment 1 as 1, and comparing the index values in the methane production stage of Experiment 2 with those of Experiment 1, the differences between the two processes can be intuitively compared, as shown in **Figure 6**.

Except for methane (CH_4) content, all other indicators in Experiment 2 were lower than those in Experiment 1. The reason may be that the raw materials were first subjected to acid treatment in the hydrogen production stage, which increased the degradation rate of cellulose, hemicellulose, lignin, and other substances. The utilization rate of metabolites in the system, including ethanol, acetic acid, pyruvic acid, butyric acid, and other organic acids, also increased accordingly.

2.4.2 Comparison of methane production rates

The methane production stage of Experiment 1 only lasted for 36 days, and the methane production reached 2557.92 mL. While the methane production stage of Experiment 2 lasted for 56 days, and the methane production only reached

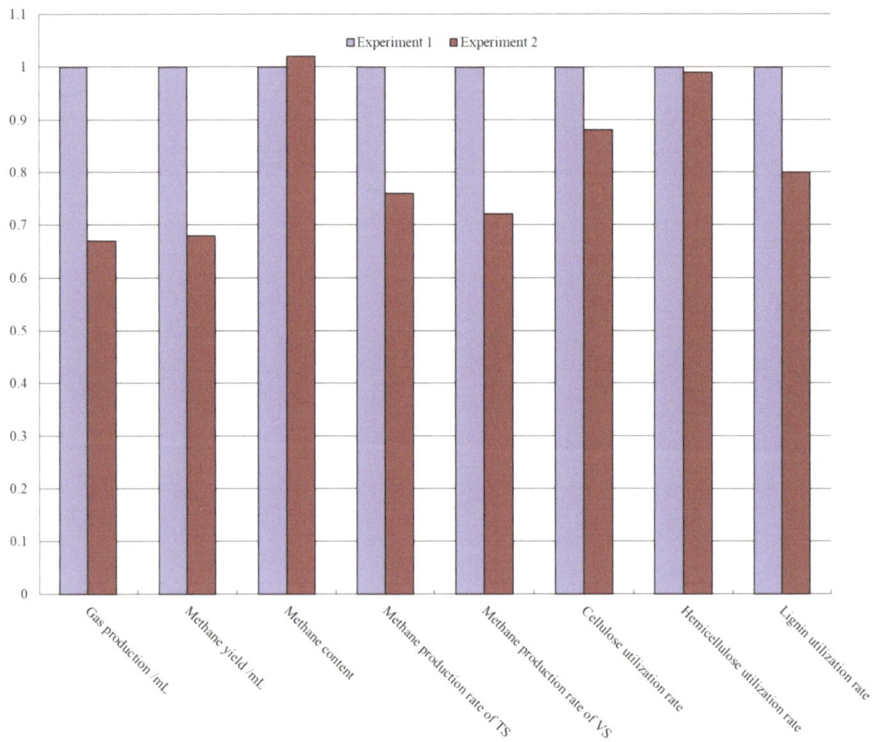

Figure 6.
Comparison of various indicators in the methane production stage.

1713.69 mL. Indicators, such as gas production volume and gas production rate, indicate that Experiment 1 has a higher utilization rate of raw materials than Experiment 2.

Thus, we calculated the methane production rate of the raw material, which can be calculated using the following formula:

$$v_n = \frac{\sum_{i=1}^{n} V_i}{V_{总}} \times 100\% \tag{1}$$

In the formula, V_n—the methane production rate of the raw material, %; V_i—methane production from the *i*th day of raw materials, mL; and $V_{总}$—total methane production of raw materials, mL.

The gas production rates of raw materials of *Eupatorium adenophorum* Spreng. in different experimental groups are shown in **Figure** 7.

From **Figure** 7, it can be seen that the initial methane production rate in Experiment 1 is lower than that in Experiment 2. Experiment 2 first ferments to produce methane, and the inoculum is activated sludge that has been domesticated in the laboratory for a long time. Among them, methanogens have higher activity and start the methane production process faster. After hydrogen-producing fermentation in Experiment 1, a large number of hydrogen-producing bacteria were enriched, and the activity of methanogens was low, manifested as a slow start of the methane production stage. After the seventh day of reaction, the methane production rate in

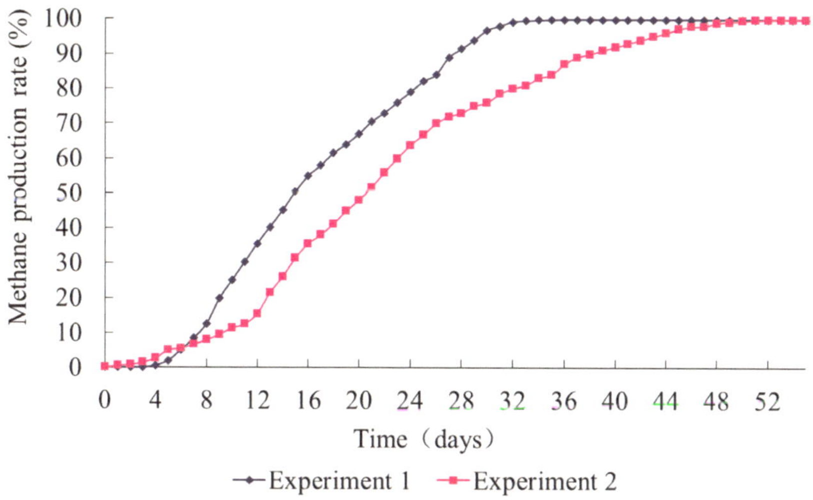

Figure 7.
Methane production rates of Experiment 1 and Experiment 2.

Experiment 1 increased significantly compared to Experiment. At the same time, the methane producing hydraulic retention time (HRT) of Experiment 1 was 36 days, which was shorter than 56 days of Experiment 2, indicating that the hydrogen production following methane producing stage is beneficial for shortening the fermentation cycle of methane production.

2.5 Analysis of energy conversion efficiency

2.5.1 Analysis of energy conversion efficiency for hydrogen and methane production

The energy utilization rate of the raw materials in this experiment can be calculated by the following formula:

$$\frac{V_{H_2} \times Q_{H_2} + V_{CH_4} \times Q_{CH_2}}{Q_{EAS} \times m_{TS}} \times 100\% \quad (2)$$

In the formula, $\mathbf{V}_{H2}$ and $\mathbf{V}_{CH4}$ are the experimental volumes (mL) of hydrogen and methane, respectively. $\mathbf{Q}_{H2}$, $\mathbf{Q}_{CH4}$, and Q_{EAS} are the combustion calorific values of hydrogen, methane, and *Eupatorium adenophorum* Spreng., respectively. The combustion calorific value of *Eupatorium adenophorum* Spreng. is 17,220 J/g [5], and m_{TS} is the experimental dry matter mass gram of *Eupatorium adenophorum* Spreng. The energy utilization efficiency at different experimental stages is shown in **Figure 8**.

From **Figure 8**, it can be seen that the energy utilization efficiency of the hydrogen production stage and methane production stage in Experiment 1 is higher than that in Experiment 2, and the experimental values of both groups are higher than the literature values [6]. The joint fermentation of hydrogen and methane production can improve energy utilization efficiency. Fermentation of first producing hydrogen and then methane can increase energy utilization efficiency by 68.54%, while fermentation of first producing methane and then hydrogen can increase energy utilization efficiency by 15.35%.

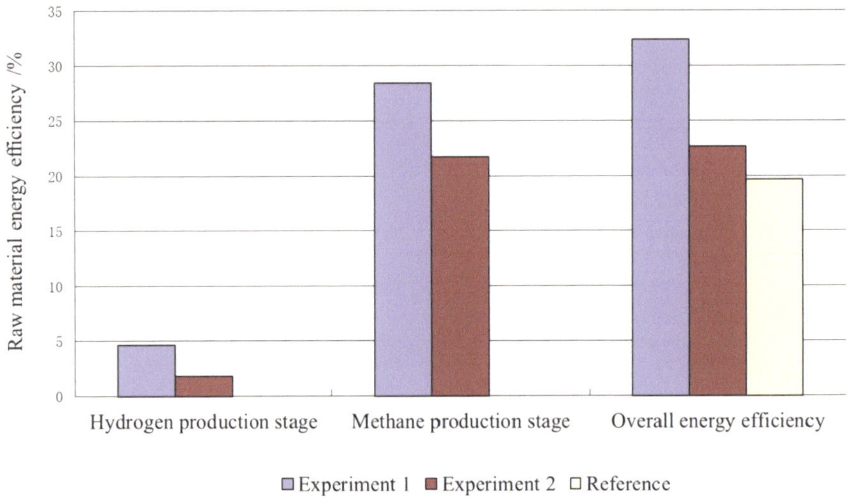

Figure 8.
Energy utilization efficiency of two experimental groups at different stages.

2.5.2 Comparison of utilization of different fermentation reaction substances and energy

For a long time, hydrogen production through fermentation from pure carbohydrates, agricultural and forestry waste straw, organic waste, and wastewater sludge has been hindered by the low calorific value per unit volume of hydrogen, resulting in low energy conversion efficiency when using biomass to produce hydrogen. In addition, fermentation to produce methane has a more effective conversion technology than fermentation to produce hydrogen, which has always been a bottleneck restricting the industrial application of fermentation to produce hydrogen [7].

However, the production of hydrogen is faster than that of methane. Experiment 1 showed that the fermentation process of producing hydrogen first and then methane was completed in 50 days, while the fermentation process of producing methane first and then hydrogen only completed the production of methane within 50 days, and continuing to produce hydrogen requires a delay of 15 days. So, joint fermentation for hydrogen production shortens the fermentation reaction cycle compared to producing methane alone or producing methane first and then hydrogen.

3. Metabolic substrates for anaerobic hydrogen and methane production

When the substrate of anaerobic digestion (carbon or carbonaceous compounds) and environmental factors (such as temperature, pH, absence of oxygen, etc.) meet specific requirements, the process of anaerobic digestion for hydrogen (H_2) and methane (CH_4) production is realized. Generally, the substrate consists of H_2, CO_2, and acetic acid as fundamental substances for metabolism.

3.1 Growth substrate for anaerobic hydrogen and methane production

As a group, methanogens can only utilize a few simple compounds, most of which are compounds containing only one carbon element (**Table 3**) [8]. The special physiological function of methanogens will result in most methanogenic bacteria in

Bacteria	Reaction	Product	$\Delta G^{O'}$ (kJ/ $molCH_4$)
Most methanogens	$4H_2$ + HCO_3^- + H^+	$CH_4 + 3H_2O$	−135
Many hydrogenotrophic methanogens	4 HCO_3^- + H^+ + H_2O	$CH_4 + 3HCO_3^-$	−145
Methanobacterium and *Methanosarcina*	$4CO + 5H_2O$	$CH_4 + 3HCO_3^- + 3H^+$	−196
Some hydrogenotrophic methanogens	$2CH_3CH_2OH$+ HCO_3^-	$2CH_3COO^- + H^+$+ $CH_4 + H_2O$	−116
Methanosarcina and *Methanothrix* spp.	$CH_3COO^- + H_2O$	$CH_4 + HCO_3^-$	−31
Methanosarcina and other methylotrophic methanogens	$4CH_3OH$	$3CH_4 + HCO_3^- + H_2O$+ H^+	−105
Methanosarcina and other methylotrophic methanogens	$4(CH_3)_3$-NH^+ + $9H_2O$	$9CH_4 + 3HCO_3^- + 4NH_4^+$+ $3H^+$	−76
Some methylotrophic methanogens	$2(CH_3)_2$-S + $3H_2O$	$3CH_4 + HCO_3^- + 2H_2S + H^+$	−49
Methanosphaera stadtmanae, methylotrophic methanogens	$CH_3OH + H_2$	$CH_4 + H_2O$	−113

Table 3.
Reactions of methanogens using different substrates.

anaerobic habitats requiring other microorganisms to provide them with substrates. Therefore, most organic matter requires the interaction of different groups of anaerobic microorganisms in the food chain in order to ultimately be converted into methane. While in an aerobic ecosystem, a single microorganism can typically completely oxidize a complex organic compound into CO_2.

The reason why methanogenic bacteria cannot convert some slightly more complex organic molecules, such as glucose, into CH_4 and CO_2 is that methanogenic bacteria cannot compete with fermentative bacteria that are more specific in utilizing complex organic molecules. The free energy of each electron in fermentative bacteria is much more negative than that in complete metabolic reactions coupled with methanogenesis or sulfate reduction, and the reaction is easier to carry out. The $\Delta G^{O'}$ of glucose fermentation conversion into acetic acid and H_2 is −27 kJ/electron, while the $\Delta G^{O'}$ of glucose complete degradation into CH_4 is only −16 kJ/electron. Therefore, a hypothetical methanogenic bacterium that utilizes glucose has to compete with more efficient fermentative bacteria (ΔG^{O} per electron is −39 kJ/electron under anaerobic bioreactor conditions). If this methanogenic bacterium converts glucose into acetic acid and CH_4, each electron in the reaction can store −42.7 kJ of free energy, but the existence of such a methanogenic bacterium has not yet been discovered [9].

From **Table 3**, it can be seen that the most common decomposition reaction of methanogens is the reduction of CO_2 to CH_4 using H_2 as a reducing agent. H_2 is the main fermentation product of anaerobic microorganisms, fungi, and protozoa. Most methanogenic bacteria (hydrotrophic type) capable of producing CH_4 from H_2-CO_2 can also use formate dehydrogenase to reduce CO_2 with formic acid as an electron donor [10]. *Methanobacterium thermoautotrophicum* and *Methanosarcina barkeri* can grow by utilizing carbon monoxide (CO) dehydrogenase to obtain electrons from CO (H_2) may be an intermediate metabolite in this reaction process [11]. Some hydrogenotrophic methanogens can also use short-chain alcohols as electron donors to oxidize secondary alcohols into ketones [12] and primary alcohols into carboxylic acids [13]. This discovery overturns the traditional view that alcohols other than methanol cannot be directly utilized by methanogens. The methanogenic bacteria *Methanosarcina* and *Methanothrix*, which are acetic acid trophic methanogens, can utilize different substrates, including methyl compounds, and sometimes H_2-CO_2 [14]. Some methylotrophic methanogenic bacterial communities, including *Methanosarcina*, *Methanococcus*, *Methanolobus*, and *Methanohalilius*, can utilize methanol and methylamine, while some cultures can also utilize methyl sulfides [15].

3.1.1 Utilizing hydrogen and carbon dioxide to produce methane

Apart from some methanogens, such as *Methanothrix* spp., which can only metabolize acetic acid, *Methanosphaera stadtmanae*, which uses hydrogen to reduce methanol, *Methanolobus tindarius*, which can only use methanol and methylamine, most methanogens can grow using hydrogen and carbon dioxide as energy sources:

$$4H_2 + CO_2 \rightarrow CH_4 + 2H_2O \quad \Delta G^{O'} = -131\ \text{kJ/mol} \tag{3}$$

In methane ecosystems, the hydrogen partial pressure is usually between 1 and 10 Pa. At this low concentration of hydrogen, the variable of free energy ($\Delta G^{O'}$) during methane production using hydrogen and carbon dioxide is −20 kJ/mol to −40 kJ/mol. In cells, the synthesis of ATP from adenosine diphosphate (ADP) and inorganic phosphates requires a minimum free energy of 50 kJ/mol. Therefore, under physiological growth conditions, less than 1 mole of ATP can be synthesized per mole of methane produced, which can serve as evidence for the coupling of methane production capacity and ADP phosphorylation through chemical permeation mechanism.

3.1.2 Production of methane through acetic acid oxidation

The degradation of acetic acid contains two reactions: the dehydrogenation of acetic acid and anaerobic oxidation of acetic acid. In the syntrophic methanogenic bacterial community (acetate-oxidizing bacteria and methanogenic archaea), the oxidation of acetic acid reaction can occur, indicating that the acetate-oxidizing bacteria first oxidize acetic acid into H_2/CO_2, and then the hydrogenotrophic methanogenic archaea convert H_2/CO_2 into methane, which is in accordance with the biochemical metabolic rules.

3.1.2.1 Acetic acid as an intermediate metabolite

The process of methane production through anaerobic digestion using hydrogen reduction involves the oxidation of sugars, peptides, lactic acid, and pyruvic acid to CO_2, or the fermentation of these organic matters to produce acetic acid and other products. These processes are generally divided into the following steps: sugar degradation to produce pyruvic acid, conversion of pyruvic acid to acetyl-CoA (coenzyme A), oxidation of acetyl-CoA to 2 molecules of CO_2 (sulfur, sulfate, and oxygen as terminal electron acceptors), or conversion of acetyl-CoA to acetic acid. When the inorganic electron acceptors, such as oxygen, nitrate, iron, magnesium, and sulfate, are lacking, these complex organic matter undergo anaerobic digestion to produce methane as the main degradation pathway, which consists of four steps: primary fermenting bacteria—hydrolyze macromolecular organic matter into amino acids,

Process	Fermentation equation	$\Delta G^{O'}$ (kJ/mol)
(1) Aceticlastic methanogenesis	$^*CH_3COO + H_2O$ — $^*CH_4 + HCO_3$	−31.0
(2) Syntrophic acetate oxidation	$^*CH_3COO + 4H_2O$— $H^*CO_3 + 4H_2 + HCO_3 + H^+$	+104.6
(3) H_2-consuming methanogenesis	$4H_2 + HCO_3 + H^+$— $CH_4 + 4H_2O$	−135.6
(4) Sum of (2) + (3)	$^*CH_3COO + H_2O$ — $H^*CO_3 + CH_4$	−31.0
(5) H_2-consuming acetogenesis	$4H_2 + 2HCO_3 + H^+$— $CH_3COO + 4H_2O$	−104.6

Table 4.
Acetic acid oxidation process.

sugars, and long-chain fatty acids; secondary fermenting bacteria (proton-reducing intertrophic bacteria)—hydrolytic products are acetic acid, hydrogen, and carbon dioxide; acetic acid hydrolysis methanogens—acetic acid degradation; and hydrogenotrophic methanogens—convert hydrogen and carbon dioxide into methane [16].

3.1.2.2 Acetic acid oxidation

The degradation of acetic acid to produce methane can be divided into two processes:

The first process is aceticlastic methanogenesis, in which acetic acid is cracked into methyl and carbonyl groups. Through biochemical reactions, the methyl group is directly converted into methane, while the carbonyl group is oxidized to carbon dioxide [17]. This reaction can occur spontaneously. Both *Methanosarcina* and *Methanosaeta* are currently known to produce methane through this reaction.

The second process contains two reactions, syntrophic acetate oxidation and hydrogenotrophic methanogenesis. This process was originally proposed by Barker [18] in 1936. In the process of syntrophic acetate oxidation, the methyl and carbonyl groups of acetic acid are oxidized to CO_2 and produce H_2 (Reaction 2 in **Table 4**). Although syntrophic acetate oxidation cannot occur spontaneously ($\Delta G^{o\prime}$ = +104.6 kJ/mol), it is accompanied by hydrogen consumption by methanogens like ethanol or fatty acid oxidation (Reaction 3 in **Table 4**) [19] ($\Delta G^{o\prime}$ = −135.6 kJ/mol), making the entire reaction process (Reaction (2) + (3)) become spontaneous ($\Delta G^{o\prime}$ = −31.0 kJ/mol) (Reaction 4 in **Table 4**) [20], which has the same stoichiometric formula with aceticlastic methanogenesis.

It can be seen that acetic acid is the most important intermediate metabolite in the process of methane production by anaerobic mineralization of organic matter.

3.2 Conclusion

The anaerobic digestion process relies on H_2, CO_2, and acetic acid as the metabolic basis. When the substrate (carbon) and environmental factors (such as temperature, pH, oxygen isolation, etc.) of anaerobic digestion can meet the system requirements, there are two ways to utilize the substrate:

1. Using hydrogen and carbon dioxide to produce methane;

$$4H_2 + CO_2 \rightarrow CH_4 + 2\,H_2O \quad \Delta G^{O'} = -131\,\text{kJ/mol} \tag{4}$$

2. There are two ways to produce methane from acetic acid oxidation and acetic acid: One is direct cracking,

$$^{*}CH_3COO^- + H_2O \rightarrow {}^{*}CH_4 + HCO_{3^-} \quad \Delta G^O = -310\ kJ/mol \tag{5}$$

The other is syntrophic acetate oxidation and hydrogenotrophic methanogenesis, accompanied by the hydrogen consumption of methanogens ($\Delta G^{O'} = -135.6$ kJ/mol), the entire reaction $\Delta G^{O'} = -31 < 0$,

$$^{*}CH_3COO^- + 4H_2O \rightarrow H^{*}CO_{3^-} + 4H_2 + HCO_{3^-} + H^+ \quad \Delta G^o = +1046\ kJ/mol \tag{6}$$

$$4H_2 + HCO_{3^-} + H^+ \rightarrow CH_4 + 4H_2O \quad \Delta G^o = -1356\ kJ/mol \tag{7}$$

$$^{*}CH_3COO^- + H_2O \rightarrow H^{*}CO_{3^-} + CH_4 \quad \Delta G^o = -310\ kJ/mol \tag{8}$$

It can be seen that the coupling of acetic acid oxidation reaction accompanied by hydrogen consumption to produce methane is the key metabolic pathway for the entire anaerobic oxidation to produce methane.

4. Symbiosis between anaerobic and methanogenic microorganisms

Anaerobic digestion is an extremely complex microbial and biochemical process. In the gradual understanding of the distribution and degradation steps of microbial communities in the anaerobic digestion process, it has been found that the most important link is substrate degradation and the interaction between different microbial communities [21]. First, substrate degradation mineralization produces methane through the oxidation of acetic acid to H_2/CO_2, which is then converted to methane. As long as the partial pressure of hydrogen in the system is maintained at a low level, energy release from the reaction can be guaranteed, and energy conservation of the system as well as stable cell growth can be sustained.

Second, neither methanogenic archaea nor hydrolytic bacteria can degrade organic matter alone, but both must be involved. Different bacterial communities live together in a compact group that is close to thermodynamic equilibrium. The evolutionary metabolic mechanism among different bacterial communities allows them to share the chemical energy of biochemical reactions among themselves. (Although the energy value released by the interaction between acetate-oxidizing bacteria and methanogenic bacteria is very low, $\Delta G^{O'} = -31.0$ kJ/mol, the two bacterial communities only share this energy of 15.5 kJ/mol for their own survival needs.) This energy deficiency will cause slow growth of bacterial communities, and they are difficult to separate from each other, even unable to survive independently after separation. This also explains why it has been difficult to achieve the separation and purification of acetic acid oxidizing bacterial systems for a long time [22]. Therefore, non-methanogenic hydrolytic bacteria and methanogenic archaea coexist, depend on each other, and constrain each other in anaerobic digestion systems. Their potential bacterial symbiosis is an important guarantee for maintaining normal life activities to achieve balance in the entire digestion process, and is a key factor to ensure the efficient degradation of hydrogen and methane production in the anaerobic digestion system [23].

In anaerobic environments, bacteria and archaea achieve methanogenesis and oxidation by interspecific electron transfer [24] (interspecific hydrogen transfer), which shuttles back and forth. In facultative intertrophic bacteria, the substrate is fermented by a single hydrolytic bacterium, while the growth of microorganisms and their metabolites is regulated by hydrogen-consuming methanogens [25]. These mutualistic bacterial communities have the following distinct characteristics:

1. Neither archaea nor bacteria can independently degrade specific organic compounds, the hydrolysis and growth of these organic compounds must involve both parties [26].

2. The distance between the syntrophic flora can affect the degradation and growth rate of organic matter, resulting in the formation of compact aggregates of bacteria and archaea.

3. The syntrophic flora live in a state close to thermal equilibrium, so the metabolism of one type of flora directly affects the metabolism of another type of flora.

4. The progressive biochemical metabolic mechanism of the syntrophic flora allows the sharing of chemical energy of biochemical reactions among the flora [27].

4.1 The culture scheme of interspecific hydrogen transfer-dependent syntrophic flora

Strict anaerobic bacteria can generate acetic acid, carbon dioxide, and hydrogen from glucose. When hydrogen partial pressure is low, from the perspective of energy balance, oxidation of nicotinamide adenine dinucleotide (NADH) and reducing ferredoxin and reduction of coupled protons are feasible, so hydrogen will be the only reduction product:

$$\text{Glucose} \rightarrow 2\ \text{acetate}^- + 2CO_2 + 4H_2 + 4H^+ \quad \Delta G^O = -216\ \text{kJ/mol} \tag{9}$$

When the fermentation bacteria (without hydrogen-consuming methanogens) are isolated and grown in pure medium, hydrogen will accumulate to a higher concentration, and then NADH oxidation will no longer occur, and sugar degradation and growth will stop. However, many fermenting bacteria can also oxidize NADH by reducing intracellular metabolites (as shown in **Table 5**).

$\Delta G^{o\prime}$, standard Gibbs free energy change expressed in kJ/mol.

The energy advantage of the coexistence of these fermentative bacteria and hydrogen-consuming methanogens in the syntrophic flora is that they can obtain more ATP. For example, when *Ruminococcus albus* grows in pure medium, it converts glucose into ethanol and produces 2 molecules of ATP. However, when *Ruminococcus albus* and hydrogen-consuming methanogens intergrow, glucose is converted into acetic acid, producing 4 molecules of ATP. Such a facultative syntrophic flora utilizes a feasible thermodynamic dynamic reaction to conserve maximum energy.

Bacteria that can oxidize NADH and produce coupled hydrogen can survive by consuming hydrogen through other anaerobic methanogens. Therefore, such fermentative bacteria, including *Synechococcus* and *Bacillus*, should be considered as specialized syntrophic flora [28]. It is possible for many fermentative bacteria that rely on low concentrations of hydrogen and formic acid to survive in methane-producing environments. However, just like other fermentative bacteria that grow rapidly, relying on the symbiotic survival of methanogenic bacteria cannot be obtained using ordinary standard enrichment and isolation methods, as shown in **Figure 9**.

Species	Reaction	$\Delta G^{o\prime}$
Ruminococcus albus	Glucose → 2 ethanol +2CO_2	−235 kJ
Selenomonas ruminantium	Glucose → 2 lactate$^-$ + 2H^+	−198 kJ
Ruminococcus flavefaciens	Glucose →acetate$^-$ + succinate^{2-} + H_2 + 3 H^+	−169 kJ
Acetobacterium woodii	Glucose → 3 acetate$^-$ + 3H^+	−311 kJ

Table 5.
H^+ reactions with NADH oxidation.

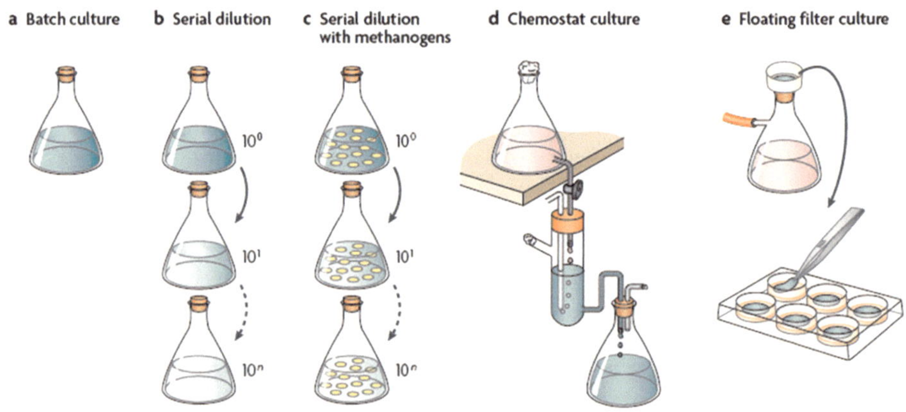

Figure 9.
Different strategies for enriching microorganisms in anaerobic environments.

The enrichment and separation operation method is as follows:

a. Batch culture, a traditional specialized medium for batch cultivation, is suitable for the enrichment and isolation of rapidly growing bacteria.

b. Serial dilution, a sequence dilution method for batch cultivation in specialized culture media, is suitable for the enrichment and isolation of a large number of bacteria, especially those coexisting with methane-producing bacteria.

c. Serial dilution with methanogens, the batch culture sequence dilution of methanogenic bacteria pregrown in a hydrogen containing substrate. Most methanogenic bacteria can effectively engulf hydrogen and formic acid and provide suitable growth conditions for bacteria that coexist with methanogenic bacteria.

d. Chemostat culture, a constant culture that enriches microorganisms with high affinity for substrates.

e. Floating filter culture, suitable for the enrichment and separation of demanding bacteria with high nutrient requirements that cannot grow on solid medium. The samples are first filtered through a 0.2-μm polycarbonate and polyester fiber membrane, and then concentrated and placed on the surface of liquid or solid medium containing carbon sources.

4.2 Symbiosis between hydrogen-producing bacteria and hydrogen-consuming methanogens

In the mutualistic microbiota, hydrogen-producing bacteria and hydrogen-consuming methanogens share redox states, affecting mutual metabolism. Under high concentration hydrogen conditions, the metabolism of hydrogen-producing bacteria is inhibited, methane metabolism is stimulated, and vice versa [29]. The transfer of metabolites between microorganisms is caused by diffusion, and the diffusion flow rate is defined by Fick's formula:

$$J = DA[(c2 - c1)/d] \tag{10}$$

In the formula, D represents the diffusion coefficient in water, A represents the surface area of the producing bacteria, C represents the concentration of metabolites, D represents the distance between two microorganisms, and J represents the flow rate of metabolites.

According to the calculations of Schink and Thauer [30], the proportion of interspecific hydrogen transfer increases significantly with cell aggregation. Anaerobic digesters and methanogens gather together to form a dense microbial community structure, similar to organs, rather than independent functional microbial suites. As early as 1936, Barker proposed the synergistic oxidation fermentation of acetic acid to produce methane and CO_2 [31], and the verification result was only observed in 1984 through the experiment of isolating the acetic acid oxidizing strain aldehyde ferredoxin oxidoreductase (AOR) from a high-temperature reactor (58°C) [32]. It also confirmed that it is a homoacetogen that can rely on hydrogen growth and reduce CO_2 to produce acetic acid [33].

Figure 10 shows the dense methanogenic particle structure, which is formed by the spontaneous aggregation of anaerobic digesters and methanogenic bacteria in an efficient methane reactor [34]. The figure is stained to show different microbial flora. Green is archaea, red is digestive bacteria and methanosaeta. The methanosaeta labeled with red and green can produce yellow fluorescence, which is easy to distinguish from bacteria.

In general, the initialization and final formation of granulation is a complex process involving physicochemical and biochemical interactions. Methane-producing sludge granulation can only be produced when the microbes are tightly packed together. The precipitation of granulation can effectively prevent microorganisms from being washed out of the reactor. The physical and mechanical damage of the granulation will lead to the serious inactivation of methanogens based on interspecific hydrogen transfer, while the activity of methanogens based on acetic acid remains unchanged. In addition, by constructing artificial aggregates or adding additional methanogens in the suspended co-culture solution, the distance between granulation is increased, and the conversion efficiency is significantly improved.

4.3 Conclusion

Since the oxidative methanogenesis of acetic acid requires the coupling of hydrogen-consuming methanogens, this shows the fact that:

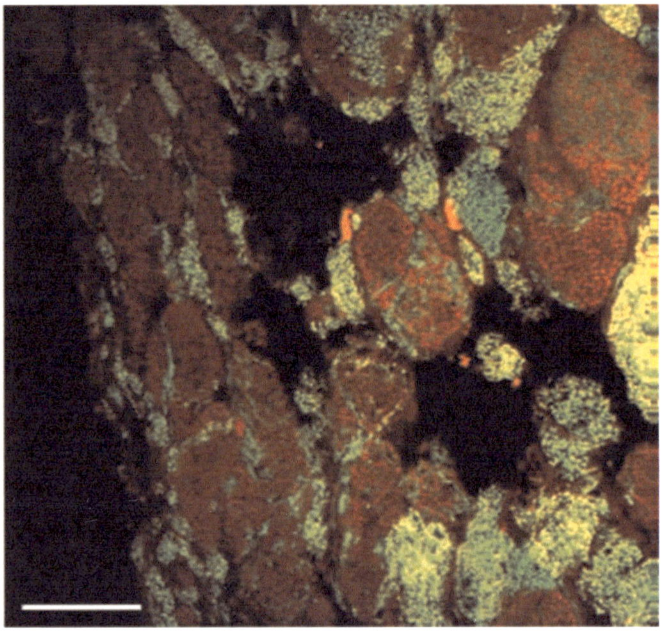

Figure 10.
Syntrophic flora of digestive bacteria and methanogenic bacteria in sludge granulation in a methanogenic bioreactor [34].

Neither hydrolytic bacteria nor methanogenic archaea can degrade organic matter alone, but both must be involved. The formation of compact aggregates by the syntrophic flora is necessary to improve the degradation rate of the substrate. The sharing of chemical energy among the syntrophic flora is necessary to meet the biochemical metabolic mechanisms.

Although the interaction between acetate-oxidizing bacteria and methanogenic bacteria results in the release of energy ($\Delta G^{O'} = -31.0$ kJ/mol), the two bacterial communities must share this energy of 15.5 kJ/mol for their own survival needs. The lack of this energy supply will cause: (1) slow growth of microbial communities—anaerobic digestion process is relatively time-consuming; (2) the formation of a mutually beneficial symbiotic coexistence—syntrophic flora that are difficult to separate, explaining that the isolation and pure cultivation of methanogenic flora are impossible.

Bacteria and archaea live together in a syntrophic way, relying on each other and constraining each other, especially between hydrogen-acetogenic bacteria and methanogenic archaea. By utilizing their mutually beneficial metabolic abilities, they overcome energy barriers and digest compounds that cannot be degraded by themselves, which is an important guarantee for maintaining normal life activities and achieving balance in the entire digestion process.

5. Energy collaborative sharing in anaerobic hydrogen and methane production processes

In the process of anaerobic digestion, even compounds that are difficult to digest can be combined with hydrogen consumption and methanogenesis ($\Delta Go' = -135.6$ kJ/mol), as long as a low hydrogen partial pressure is maintained in the fermentation

DOI: http://dx.doi.org/10.5772/intechopen.1007305

system and the reduction equivalent is transferred by the component of interspecific electron transfer (interspecific hydrogen transfer) shuttling back and forth. Although the process of acetic acid oxidation and hydrogen consumption to produce methane is achieved by acetic acid oxidizing bacteria and hydrogenotrophic methanogenic bacteria, the result of their interaction is the release of energy, but the energy value is very low ($\Delta G^{0\prime} = -31.0$ kJ/mol). At the same time, the two types of bacteria must share this energy value for their own survival needs. Insufficient supply of this energy will cause the slow growth of mutualistic bacterial communities, and form strict mutually beneficial symbiotic coexistence that is difficult to separate from each other, making it impossible for them to live independently after separation. This also explains why it has long been difficult, or even impossible, to achieve the separation and purification of a mixed culture system for the oxidation of syntrophic acetic acid.

As early as the 1940s, Russian microbiologist Vasily L. Omelianski proposed that ethanol is an excellent methanogenic hydrogen producing substrate. Subsequently, Professor Albert Barker from the University of California, USA, continued to study the utilization of ethanol for methane production and the biochemical metabolic mechanisms of methane production, and named this methane-producing bacterium *Methanobacillus omelianskii* [35]. The study also found that during methane production, the *Methanobacillus omelianskii* strain uses ethanol as an electron acceptor to reduce carbon dioxide. In the absence of carbon dioxide, this strain oxidizes ethanol and releases hydrogen until thermodynamic equilibrium [36]. In 1967, Marvin P. Bryant's [37] research group at the University of Illinois in the United States conducted experiments showing that *Methanobacillus omelianskii* is a mixed culture consisting of S-organisms and MoH methane-producing strains. The S-organisms ferment ethanol to produce acetic acid and hydrogen, which is then utilized by the MoH strain to achieve optimal thermodynamic equilibrium and promote their growth. Then, M. J. Wolin of the same research group theorized that the stress effect of hydrogen formation mechanism is related to the change of the free energy of chemical reaction equilibrium $NADH + H^+ \rightarrow NAD^+ + H_2$, which is conducive to the formation of hydrogen only under the condition of low partial pressure of hydrogen. In 1985, Professor J.G. Zeikus of Michigan State University proposed a co-culture system of *Methanosarcina barkeri* and *Desulfovibrio vulgaris*. With ethanol or acetic acid as the growth substrate providing carbon source and energy, the sulfate reduction of *Desulfovibrio vulgaris* is coupled with interspecific hydrogen transfer, and hydrogen as an electron acceptor participates in the reduction of sulfate and reduces methanogenesis. Although this is not a conventional mutuotrophic synergistic metabolic effect, it also illustrates that the loss of a potential electron acceptor for methanogenesis can be a competitive mechanism to reduce its methanogenic potential [30].

5.1 H_2 hypothesis theory

In 1970, American biologist Lynn Margulis published a book "*The Origin of Eukaryotes*," in which she proposed that aerobic bacteria are engulfed by amoeba-like prokaryotes and consume long-term symbiotic energy to become mitochondria, blue-green algae are engulfed and consume symbiotic energy to become chloroplasts, and spirochetes are engulfed and consume symbiotic energy to become primitive flagella. Subsequently, the endosymbiotic hypothesis [38] has been popularized, stating that mitochondria originate from bacteria, meaning that bacteria are engulfed by eukaryotes and evolve into mitochondria over a long period of symbiosis. This theory suggests that the ancestral promitochondria (a Gram-negative bacterium that undergoes tricarboxylic acid (TCA) cycling and electron transfer) are engulfed by prokaryotes and form a symbiotic relationship with the host. In this symbiotic relationship, both the symbiote and the host gain: the promitochondria can obtain more nutrients from the host, while the host can borrow the oxidative decomposition function of the promitochondria to obtain more energy.

The traditional theory of mitochondrial origin holds that for the host, the benefit of mitochondria is to degrade hydrocarbons through respiration to increase ATP production efficiency. However, the premise of accepting this view is to accept the following hypotheses: (1) The host cannot synthesize enough ATP on its own. (2) Symbionts produce far more ATP than they need. (3) Symbionts can export ATP to the surrounding environment, so that the host can feel this benefit. Most archaea are strictly dependent on hydrogen to produce ATP [39]. In addition, H_2O and CO_2 are both energy and carbon sources for most inorganic autotrophic methanogens, and only a few methanogens can use alternative carbon sources, such as methylamine, formic acid, and acetic acid (all of which are metabolites of eubacteria), and a very small number can be grown in a separate acetic acid substrate [40]. For methanogens, the three anaerobic metabolites of the symbiotic organism (CO_2, H_2, and acetate) provide energy for their growth. In addition, methanogens coupled with hydrogen-producing hydrogenase and independently living non-symbiotic eubacteria are strictly anaerobic. Under such hypothetical conditions, a symbiotic system is formed between eubacteria (symbiote) capable of independent survival, producing H_2 and CO_2, and methanogenic archaea (host). They should satisfy an anaerobic environment where there are enough CO_2 and environmental H_2 (geological H_2) that the host methanogens are able to survive from the start, as shown in **Figure 11(a)**.

If the environmental H_2 of the symbiotic system is removed due to physical factors (regardless of how), the host immediately transforms into heterotrophic symbionts—eubacteria—to survive, as shown in **Figure 11(b)**. There are two states: (1) the host tightly adheres to the symbiont and (2) the host benefits the most from the symbiotic connector. It can be imagined that the larger the surface area of the host cell, the more it can envelop the symbiote (archaea do not contain a cytoskeleton and do not undergo phagocytosis), allowing more H_2 and CO_2 to enter through the host cell fluid. A single input substrate cannot meet the needs of the host to meet the requirements of the symbiotic organism. The input carbon metabolism flows in different directions. First, the host's hydrocarbon metabolism must gradually improve its regulatory properties to move backward (a sequence of evolutionary processes). Second, the hydrocarbon metabolism of the symbiotic organism must first be transferred to the cell fluid and then transferred through endosymbiotic gene transfer (single reset of existing components). The two carbon metabolism pathways flow in opposite directions (catabolism and synthetic assimilation) in the same cell fluid. Only by abandoning the host's metabolic pathway can the symbiotic organism survive, as shown in **Figure 11 (d)**. The hydrogen hypothesis theory explains a fundamental eukaryotic cell lifestyle different from those previously proposed. First, it is believed that the origin of heterotrophic organs (symbionts) is the same as that of eukaryotic cell populations. Second, there are three requirements for the host methanogens: (1) anaerobic, (2) strictly dependent on H_2 metabolism, and (3) strictly autotrophic.

The H_2 hypothesis theory tells us that:

Most archaea rely heavily on H_2 to produce ATP, while H_2O and CO_2 are both their sources of energy and carbon. Only a few methanogens can utilize alternative carbon sources, such as methylamine, formic acid, and acetic acid (all of which are

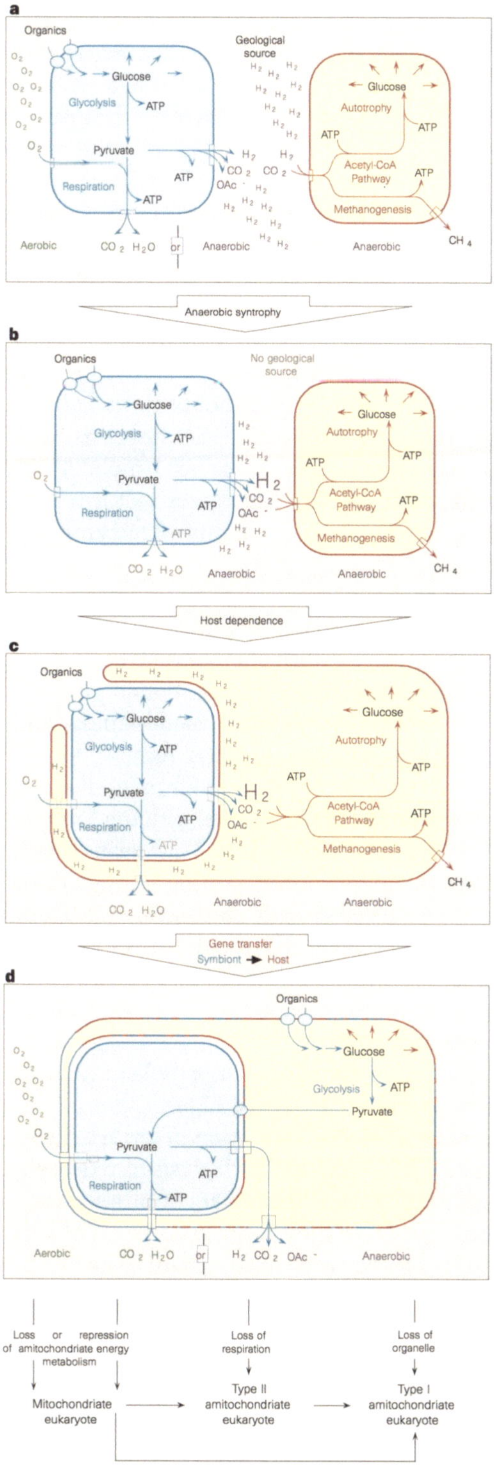

Figure 11.
Symbiotic system between eubacteria- producing H_2 and CO_2 and methanogenic archaea [27].

metabolites of eubacteria), and a very small number can grow in a separate acetic acid substrate. For methanogens, the three anaerobic metabolites (CO_2, H_2, and acetate) of the symbiotic system provide energy for their growth. The anaerobic mutualism between methanogens and hydrogen-producing organisms has been confirmed [41], and the endosymbiotic methanogens are dependent on hydrogenase particles in the cytoplasm [42].

5.2 ATP energy mechanism of anaerobic digestion microbial community

Due to the low energy involved in anaerobic metabolism, the symbiotic microbial communities are experts in "minimizing" energy utilization. As a universal energy source for cellular metabolism, ATP synthesis requires +32 kJ/mol under standard conditions, while in the assumed [ATP] = 10 mM, [ADP] = 1 mM, and [P_i] = 10 mM cell growth environment, it requires +50 kJ/mol [43]. In addition, the thermal reaction steps in the total energy budget always experience heat loss, which is inevitable during the metabolic process. The estimated heat loss per 1 mole of ATP synthesized is about 20 kJ/mol. Therefore, the entire metabolic process requires 70 kJ/mol to synthesize 1 mole of ATP, which is the lowest energy required to synthesize 1 mole of ATP in known metabolic processes [44].

Under normal physiological conditions, a change in free energy from −60 kJ to −70 kJ requires phosphorylation of 1 mole of ADP to 1 mole of ATP. This energy does not require an energy-level gradient, just like the formation of ATP through substrate-level phosphorylation, but can be transported by membrane-bound protons for redox reactions or other exothermic reactions, including relying on membrane-bound ATP synthase to drive ATP synthesis to achieve small quantum reactions. Assumptions have been made regarding the ratio of three-proton transport required to form each molecule of ATP, although studies have shown that this stoichiometry varies with the formation or hydrolysis of three to five protons in each ATP molecule [27]. This means that free energy changes in the range of 15–25 kJ (equivalent to a proton passing through the cell membrane), maintaining energy balance and cell growth. As described in **Table 6**, these values are characteristic values for bacteria converting propionate or butyrate [45].

$\Delta G^{o\prime}$, standard Gibbs free energy expressed in kJ/mol, H partial pressure expressed in 1 Pa, CH and CO partial pressures expressed in 104 Pa, and other compound concentrations expressed in 10 mM.

The propionate and butyrate conversion metabolism caused by syntrophic bacillus and monas, respectively, is shown in **Figure 12**.

During the metabolic process, the formation of oxidized coenzyme A esters in cellular tissues consumes ATP, while the hydrolysis of oxidized coenzyme A esters in cellular tissues produces ATP. In the metabolism of propionate, the decarboxylation of oxaloacetate to pyruvate can drive the energy absorption of acetyl-CoA to methylmalonyl CoA [46]. The conversion of malate to oxaloacetate in propionate metabolism and the oxidation of hydroxybutyryl CoA in butyrate metabolism both rely on NADH reactions, while the oxidative coupling of NADH from ferredoxin to hydrogenase produces hydrogen. So far, no NADH-dependent hydrogenase gene has been found in the obtained genome sequences of syntrophic bacterial communities. From an energy perspective, the oxidation of succinate in propionate metabolism to fumarate and butyryl CoA in butyrate metabolism to crotonyl CoA are the most difficult steps. Even at a hydrogen partial pressure of 1 Pa (the lowest hydrogen partial pressure required to maintain the survival of methanogens), these reactions are also energy-absorbing reactions. To drive these reactions, a metabolic energy called

Reaction	$\Delta G^{o\prime}$	$\Delta G'$ (at 1 Pa H_2)
Proton-reducing bacteria		
$Propionate^- + 2H_2O \rightarrow acetate^- + 3H_2$	+72 kJ	–21 kJ
$Butyrate^- + 2H_2O \rightarrow 2\ acetate^- + H^+ + 2H_2$	+48 kJ	–22 kJ
Methanogens		
$4H_2 + CO_2 \rightarrow CH_4 + 2H_2O$	−131 kJ	–15 kJ
$Acetate^- + H^+ \rightarrow CO_2 + CH_4$	−36 kJ	–36 kJ

Table 6.
Energy characteristic values of syntrophic flora.

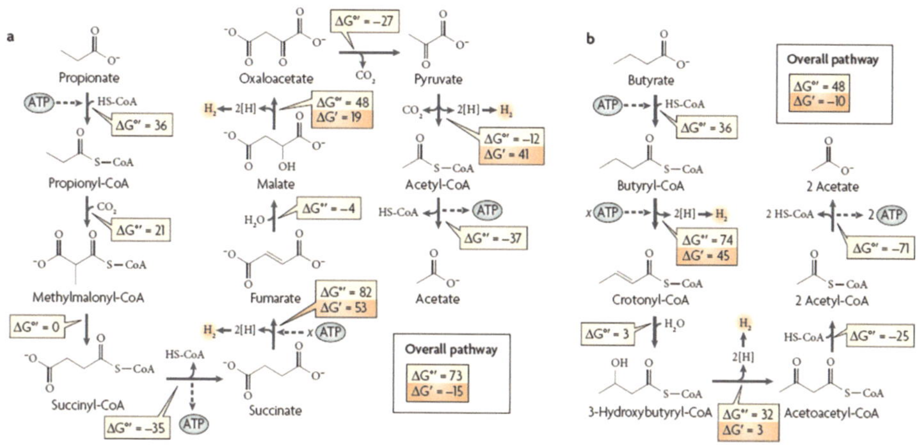

Figure 12.
Biochemical metabolic pathways of syntrophic propionate and butyrate oxidation (a means propionate oxidation, b means butyrate oxidation, the unit values of $\Delta G^{o\prime}$ and $\Delta G'$ (at 1 Pa H_2) for each metabolic reaction are kJ/mol, and the reduction equivalent values in the oxidation reaction are [H])

"Reverse Electron Transport" needs to be inputted. The metabolic mechanism for the oxidation of succinic acid to fumarate ($E^{o\prime}$ = +33 mV) in a syntrophic bacterial growth system is highly likely to be similar to the energy conversion mechanism of fumarate respiration in *Wolinella succinogenes*, but the actual situation is opposite. *Bacillus subtilis* can also utilize reverse electron transfer to oxidize succinic acid and simultaneously couple with methyl naphthoquinone for reduction ($E^{o\prime}$ = –80 mV) [47]. Methyl naphthoquinone binds to cytochrome b on the outer side of the cell membrane, and when reduced methyl naphthoquinone is oxidized in the cytoplasm between membranes, it forms protons that move inward. In the syntrophic propionate metabolism system, the oxidation of methyl naphthoquinone is linked to membrane-bound hydrogenases or formate dehydrogenases. The oxidation of succinate to fumarate requires a proton gradient across the membrane, and ATP is required to ensure the formation of hydrogen or formic acid outside the plasma membrane. In a syntrophic system, methanogens consume the hydrogen and formic acid produced in the system. When hydrogenase is specifically used to reduce protons located in the intermembrane cytoplasm, formate dehydrogenase in the cytoplasm produces formic acid. The membrane-bound methyl naphthoquinone complex enzyme allows electrons to shuttle back and forth between hydrogenase and formate dehydrogenase, achieving succinate oxidation. This hypothesis enables enzyme complexes to convert ATP into hydrogen and formic acid (**Figure 13**).

The widely accepted view is that regardless of bacterial or mitochondrial membranes, hydrolysis of one molecule of ATP will result in three protons passing through the membrane structure [48]. Therefore, the smallest energy unit that living cells in the body can utilize is no longer the unit structure of ATP, but the proton carrier in the form of mass energy conversion, which obtains one-third of the energy equivalent to ATP units during the process of crossing the cell membrane. It can be considered that the minimum reaction free energy value at the disposal of microbial cells in metabolic reactions is −20 kJ/mol, which is the minimum energy requirement for microbial communities to survive on their own in the process of mutualistic symbiosis metabolism.

5.3 Energy conversion of hydrogen and methane production in the syntrophic process

5.3.1 Hydrogen production depends on hydrogenase and ferredoxin

Although hydrogen is not abundant in nature, it plays a crucial role in microbial metabolism [49]. Some microorganisms can continuously produce and consume hydrogen because they contain hydrogenases, which can reversibly convert hydrogen into protons and electrons. Anaerobic microorganisms use protons as terminal electron acceptors to oxidize organic matter and produce hydrogen [50]. Although the generation of hydrogen is a simple redox reaction, it requires the participation of enzymes with complex reactive centers. The midpoint redox value of the redox couple H_2/H^+ ($E^{0'}$ = −414 mV) is lower than that of O_2/H_2O ($E^{0'}$ = +818 mV). By comparing, the midpoint redox value of O_2/H_2O is 1.2 V higher, which is important for aerobic respiration. However, from the energy perspective, it is difficult to use the electron transfer intermediate $NADH/FADH_2$ (flavin adenine dinucleotide) to reduce protons with a lower midpoint redox value of H_2/H^+. The midpoint redox values $E^{0'}$ of NAD^+/NADH and $FADH/FADH_2$ are −320 and − 220 mV, respectively. Another common electron transfer intermediate is ferredoxin, whose redox value $E^{0'}$ of $Fd_{(ox)}/Fd_{(red)}$ is −398 mV, or even lower. In the reaction of converting pyruvate into acetic

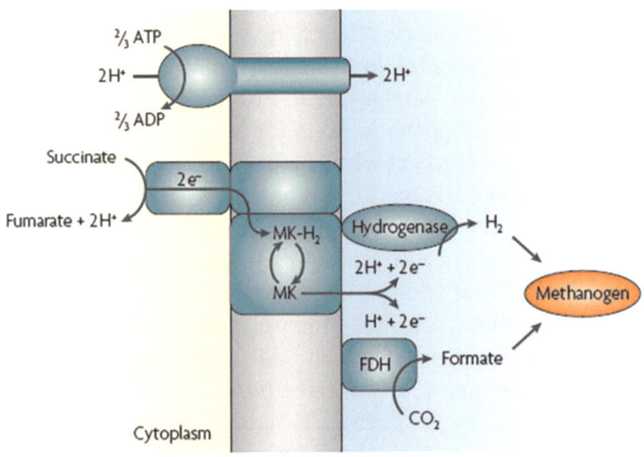

Figure 13.
Possible biochemical metabolic mechanism of reverse electron transfer for the oxidation of succinate to fumarate.

acid and carbon dioxide, ferredoxin is a key electron transfer intermediate and an intermediate step in the metabolic process of strictly anaerobic bacteria (such as *Clostridium*) [33].

$$\text{Pyruvate}^- + H^+ + HS - CoA + 2Fd(ox) \rightarrow \text{acetyl} - CoA + CO_2 + 2Fd\ (red)\Delta G^{O'} = -22\ kJ/mol \quad (11)$$

The conversion of acetyl-CoA to acetic acid is coupled with the synthesis of ATP by substrate-level phosphorylation, and the oxidation of reducing ferredoxin is coupled with the reduction of protons, and is an energy release process. Therefore, in the pure culture of anaerobic microorganisms, accompanied by pyruvate fermentation and growth, a large amount of hydrogen can be produced [51].

Facultative anaerobic bacteria, like *Escherichia coli* and *Enterobacter aerogenes*, *Shewanella oneidensis* and *Citrobacter freundii* [52], use pyruvate formase to convert pyruvate during fermentation.

$$\text{Pyruvate}^- + HS - CoA \rightarrow \text{acetyl} - CoA + \text{formate}^- \quad \Delta G^{o'} = -16\ kJ/mol \quad (12)$$

Formic acid is converted to hydrogen by formate hydrogenase (a membrane connective enzyme complex) [53]. In terms of energy conversion, hydrogen produced by formate hydrogenase is similar to hydrogen produced by ferredoxin intermediates, as shown in **Table** 7.

In methanogenic syntrophic bacterial systems, energy balance is critical for the oxidation of NADH, especially the oxidation of $FADH_2$ and the reduction of coupled protons [54]. Methanogens consume hydrogen to reduce the partial pressure of hydrogen, and this conversion reaction releases energy so that proton reduction can be achieved, and energy balance is maintained. There are also many methanogens that use hydrogen to reduce carbon dioxide, and here it is necessary to strictly distinguish whether methanogens contain cytochrome b [55]. Methanogens, which do not contain cytochrome b, use the electron transport intermediate-ferredoxin and the F_{420} factor ($E^{0'}$ $F_{420}/F_{420}H_2$ = 357 mV). These methanogens consume low concentrations of hydrogen and are the most important hydrogen scavengers in the syntrophic flora.

Reaction	**$\Delta G^{o'}$**	**$\Delta G'$ (at 1 Pa H_2)**
Hydrogen formation by anaerobic bacteria		
$2\ Fd_{(red)} + 2\ H^+ \rightarrow 2\ Fd_{(ox)} + H_2$	+3 kJ	–26 kJ
$Formate^- + H^+ \rightarrow CO_2 + H_2$	−3 kJ	–32 kJ
$NADH + H^+ \rightarrow NAD^+ + H_2$	+18 kJ	−11 kJ
$FADH_2 \rightarrow FAD + H_2$	+37 kJ	+8 kJ
Hydrogen consumption by methanogens		
$H_2 + F_{420} \rightarrow F_{420} - H_2$	–11 kJ	+18 kJ
$H_2 + 2\ Fd_{(ox)} \rightarrow 2\ Fd_{(red)}$	−3 kJ	+26 kJ

Table 7.
Energy of intracellular redox reactions.

5.3.2 Methane production depends on H_2 and hydrogen-consuming bacteria

The conversion of complex organic macromolecules (such as cellulose) into methane and carbon dioxide in natural habitats requires the synergistic action of four different microbial communities, namely, primary hydrolytic bacteria, secondary hydrolytic bacteria, and two types of methanogens. The degree of interdependence of these microbial communities varies greatly depending on the type of bacteria. Like the food chain, secondary organisms always depend on and use primary organisms as substrates, and also exert influence on primary metabolites by removing primary metabolites. The polymers (polysaccharides, proteins, nucleic acids, lipids, etc.) are first converted into oligomers and monomers (sugars, amino acids, purines, pyrimidines, fatty acids, and glycerol) under the action of extracellular hydrolases, which are hydrolyzed by primary fermentation bacteria and further convert the monomers into fatty acids, succinic acid, lactic acid, ethanol, etc. In these hydrolytic fermentation products, acetic acid, H_2, CO_2, and other carbon compounds can be converted into methane and carbon dioxide by methanogenic bacteria. For other fermentation products (such as fatty acids with more than two carbons, ethanol with more than one atom of carbon, branched chain, or aromatic fats), hydrolysis is required by other fermenting bacteria, so-called secondary hydrolytic bacteria (specialized subreductants), which convert the substrate into acetic acid, carbon dioxide, hydrogen, and formic acid, the latter of which is used by methanogens to produce methane. Under the action of methanogenesis, the degradation function of primary fermentation bacteria is exerted through the oxidation of hydrophilic bacteria, the end of the degradation chain. When the hydrogen partial pressure is lower than 10 Pa, the electrons of NADH reoxidation potential (−320 mV) are released in the form of H_2 molecules, so that the fermentation products are more converted into acetic acid, CO_2, and H_2, rather than into ethanol and butyrate. In this way, more ATP can also be produced. The process takes the fermentation reaction of hexose by *Clostridium butyricum* as an example [56].

$$\begin{gathered}\text{Glucose} + 2H_2O \rightarrow 0.7\ \text{butyrate} + 0.6\ \text{acetate} + 1.3H^+ + 2CO_2 + 2.6H_2 \\ \Delta G^{O'} = -233\ \text{kJ/mol (each molecule of glucose produces 3.3 molecules of ATP)}\end{gathered} \quad (13)$$

When $[H_2]$ = 10 Pa, the entire reaction becomes:

Glucose + $2H_2O \rightarrow$ 2 acetate + $2H^+$ + $2CO_2$ + $4H_2$ $\Delta G^{O'} = -280$ kJ/mol (each molecule of glucose produces 4 molecules of ATP, of which 2 molecules are from glycolysis and 2 molecules from the acetokinase reaction).

It can be seen that in order to ensure the 70 kJ/mol required for ATP synthesis and obtain the best energy utilization path, the bacteria will make a trade-off choice whether to maintain a low hydrogen partial pressure according to the substrate conditions.

In a normal anoxic sediment system containing a hydrophilic active community and maintaining a low hydrogen partial pressure, the pathway of carbon flow and electron flow is the "peripheral" pathway. In comparison, the role of the pathway of fermentation intermediate metabolites in the "intermediate" pathway is not very significant. However, the role of the "intermediate" pathway is not useless, as the lipids and amino acids in the fermentation raw material always produce fatty acids during the fermentation process, and once any situation occurs that triggers an increase in the amount of hydrogen in the system (for example, excessive fermentation substrate is used to inhibit methanogenesis, resulting in a decrease in pH < 6.0, or the production of certain toxic compounds), the "intermediate" metabolite pathway is very important. When the amount of fatty acids in the system increases, it will cause a decrease in pH value and inhibit the occurrence of hydrogenotrophic methane production. In this case, the final result will be a "flip" of the entire system, which means that as a large amount of odorous fatty acids accumulate, the fermentation methane production will completely stop, just like the situation in an unbalanced anaerobic sludge digester. It can be seen that in the entire process of methane production, the hydrogenotrophic methanogenic bacterial community plays the most basic role as a flow regulator, while the syntrophic fatty acid hydrolytic oxidation flora is affected by whether there is residual hydrogen in the system that has not been removed by hydrogenotrophic methanogenic bacteria in a timely manner.

Homoacetogens (⑤ in **Figure 14**) not only convert one carbon compound and hydrogen into acetic acid during the degradation process, but also participate in the fermentation of sugars and the degradation of special substrates, such as N-methyl compounds and methylphenol. In certain low pH and low-temperature environments, it can also complete the methanogenic reaction with hydrogenophilic methanogens.

5.3.3 Energy conversion in hydrogen and methane production processes

Compared with aerobic degradation or anaerobic respiration, anaerobic methane production process releases the least amount of energy. From hexose to methane and carbon dioxide, the energy released by anaerobic process is only equivalent to 15% of the energy released by aerobic process [57].

$$C_6H_{12}O_6 + 6O_2 \rightarrow 6CO_2 + 6H_2O \quad \Delta G^{O'} = -2870 \text{ kJ/mol} \tag{14}$$

$$C_6H_{12}O_6 \rightarrow 3CO_2 + 3CH_4 \quad \Delta G^{O'} = -390 \text{ kJ/mol} \tag{15}$$

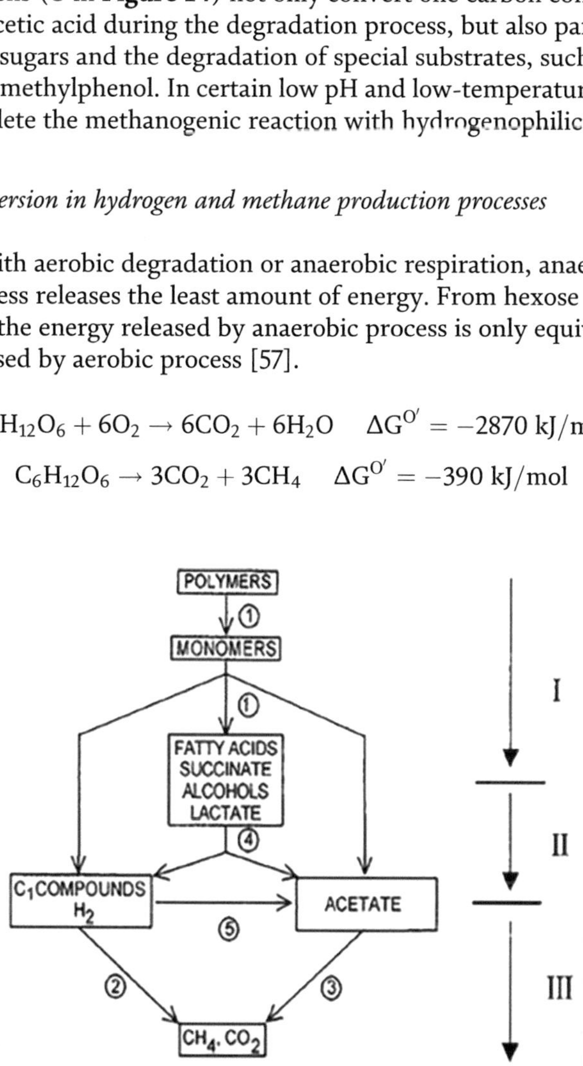

FIG. 1. Carbon and electron flow through the various trophic groups of microorganisms involved in the methanogenic degradation of complex organic matter in an anoxic freshwater habitat. Groups of bacteria involved: 1, primary fermenting bacteria; 2, hydrogen-oxidizing methanogens; 3, acetate-cleaving methanogens; 4, secondary-fermenting ("syntrophic") bacteria; 5, homoacetogenic bacteria. I, II, and III, steps in degradation. Based on reference 144; modified from reference 95.

Figure 14.
Carbon and electron flow pathways in anaerobic digestion process.

From the equation, it can be seen that compared with other oxidative degradation processes, anaerobic digestion methane production releases lower energy, which explains why methane production occurs only when other electron acceptors have been reduced, and methane is the last product of the carbon cycle. The digestion process produces such a small amount of energy that the result is that methane, as a reaction product, stores a significant portion of the energy value equivalent to that available during the degradation of oxygen-consuming biomass. This energy can be utilized under subsequent aerobic conditions, that is, what we call the use of its thermal or physicochemical energy as an energy substance.

The energy value released by methanogenic transformation is low, requiring the microorganisms involved in the transformation process to collaborate in an efficient manner. Under the condition of limited energy supply, if one of the interdependent hydrolytic bacteria and archaea does not participate in the reaction, the other will not be able to complete the reaction. The combination of the two shows an indispensable metabolic pattern, and we also call such a synergistic effect as mutuotrophic symbiosis. Two different microorganisms are interdependent and synergistic when degrading a certain substrate due to energy reasons. In such a symbiotic organism, in order to maintain efficient synergies, it is objectively required that the amount of material shuttling back and forth between them be kept at a low level (**Table 8**).

5.4 Evaluation of energy conversion efficiency for joint production of hydrogen and methane

The processes of anaerobic digestion, such as hydrolysis stage, hydrogen and acid production stage, and methane production stage, are essentially the organic coupling of hydrogen production and methane production. First, the hydrogen and acid production stage is the process in which various water-soluble products obtained from the hydrolysis stage are further decomposed and metabolized by hydrogen and acid-

Reaction	$\Delta G^{0\prime}$ (kJ/mol)
Hydrogen-releasing reactions	
$CH_3CH_2OH^- + H_2O \rightarrow CH_3COO^- + H^+ + 2H_2$	+9.6 kJ
$CH_3CH_2CH_2\,COO^- + 2H_2O \rightarrow 2CH_3COO^- + 2H^+ + 2H_2$	+48.3 kJ
$CH_3CH_2COO^- + 2H_2O \rightarrow CH_3COO^- + CO_2 + 3H_2$	+76.0 kJ
$CH_3COO^- + 2H_2O + H^+ \rightarrow 2CO_2 + 4H_2$	+94.9 kJ
$CH_3CH(CH_3)CH_2COO^- + CO_2 + 2H_2O \rightarrow 3CH_3COO^- + 2H^+ + H_2$	+25.2 kJ
Hydrogen-consuming reactions	
$4H_2 + 2CO_2 \rightarrow CH_3COO^- + H^+ + 2H_2O$	−94.9 kJ
$4H_2 + CO_2 \rightarrow CH_4 + 2H_2O$	−131.0 kJ
$H_2 + S^0 \rightarrow H_2S$	−33.9 kJ
$4H_2 + SO_4^{2-} + H^+ \rightarrow HS + 4H_2O$	−151.0 kJ
$H_2C(NH_3^+)COO^- + H_2 \rightarrow CH_3COO^- + 2NH_4^+$	−78.0 kJ
Fumarate + $H_2 \rightarrow$ succinate	−86.0 kJ

Table 8.
Reaction equations of hydrogen and methane production in syntrophic process.

producing bacteria to form substrates for methane-producing bacteria [4]. The products mainly include acetic acid, hydrogen, and carbon dioxide. Second, the hydrogen production process provides substrates and energy for methane production. The methane production process consumes hydrogen, reduces hydrogen partial pressure, and enables the hydrogen production process to proceed normally. However, the process of hydrogen fermentation often involves the production of a large amount of carbon dioxide, resulting in a significant loss of carbon sources in the system, which is also unfavorable for energy recovery.

5.4.1 Energy conversion efficiency of hydrogen and methane production separately

Yang Bin from Yunnan Normal University [58] calculated the energy conversion efficiency of anaerobic digestion systems for producing hydrogen and methane separately.

The energy conversion efficiency of methanogenic fermentation is not high (see Table 5.7) [59], which is not only related to the low utilization rate of raw materials and the narrow range of substrates that can be directly utilized, but also due to the fact that the important energy gas H2 produced during methane fermentation is not recovered and utilized, but is instead utilized by hydrogen-phagocytic methanogens and converted into CH_4 ($4H_2 + 2CO_2 \rightarrow CH_4 + 2H_2O$). For every 1 mol of methane produced, 4 mol of hydrogen is consumed, resulting in an energy loss of 169.2 kJ/mol (**Table 9**).

For hydrogen-producing fermentation, due to the accumulation of propionic acid and butyric acid, the fermentation of raw materials is incomplete, and part of raw materials will be left, and small molecular organic acids, such as acetic acid, propionic acid, and butyric acid, in the fermentation products and alcohols will not be further utilized and remain in the hydrogen-producing fermentation liquid, resulting in the energy contained in these organic substances not being converted into a certain form. As a result, the energy conversion efficiency of hydrogen-producing fermentation is low, which has been confirmed by many scholars [60]. In conventional anaerobic digestion, because the hydrogen produced by fermentation can be quickly utilized by hydrogen-phagocytic methanogens and converted into CH_4, the hydrogen partial pressure can be kept very low in the environment, so that the intermediate product of fermentation is mainly acetic acid. However, for hydrogen-producing fermentation, because the activity of methanogens that can use hydrogen is inhibited, the generated hydrogen is easy to accumulate, resulting in higher hydrogen partial pressure, so that the above-mentioned reaction cannot proceed to the right, and the electrons generated in the process of glycolysis will accumulate in the intermediate products, thus forming reductive products, such as propionic acid, butyric acid, and ethanol.

Fermentation raw materials	Theoretical efficiency of energy conversion (%)	Actual efficiency of energy conversion (%)
Corn stalks	65.55	32.78
Wheat straw	61.14	30.58
Straw	64.05	32.02
Pig manure	65.56	32.80

Table 9.
Energy conversion efficiency of methane production from common raw materials.

Propionic acid and butyric acid can cause toxic effects on hydrogen-producing fermentation, inhibit the progress of hydrogen-producing fermentation, and lead to incomplete hydrogen-producing fermentation [61].

As shown in **Figure 15**, when fermenting bacteria perform glycolysis, different products will be generated due to the difference in the partial pressure of hydrogen in the environment. Carbohydrates initially convert hexose to pyruvate via the Embden-Meyerhof-Parnas (EMP) pathway and release hydrogen, which is then transferred to the carrier NAD^+ to become NADH. Under anaerobic conditions, NADH is restored to NAD^+ by generating molecular hydrogen, i.e. $NADH + H^+ \leftarrow \rightarrow NAD^+ + H_2$. However, the free energy of this reaction in the standard state is $\triangle G^0 = +18$ kJ, so the reaction is thermodynamically unfavorable. In order for the reaction to proceed smoothly to the right, the partial pressure of hydrogen must be reduced. It can be seen from the calculation that when the partial pressure of hydrogen drops to 10^{-4} atm, the reaction free energy of the above-mentioned reaction will be less than zero, and then the reaction may proceed to the right [62].

5.4.2 *Quantitative relationship of energy conversion for joint production of hydrogen and methane*

Hallenbeck [63] and Benemann [64] quantitatively described the basic principles and energy conversion relationships of hydrogen and methane production in anaerobic digestion. Hydrogen production is accompanied by the generation of intermediate

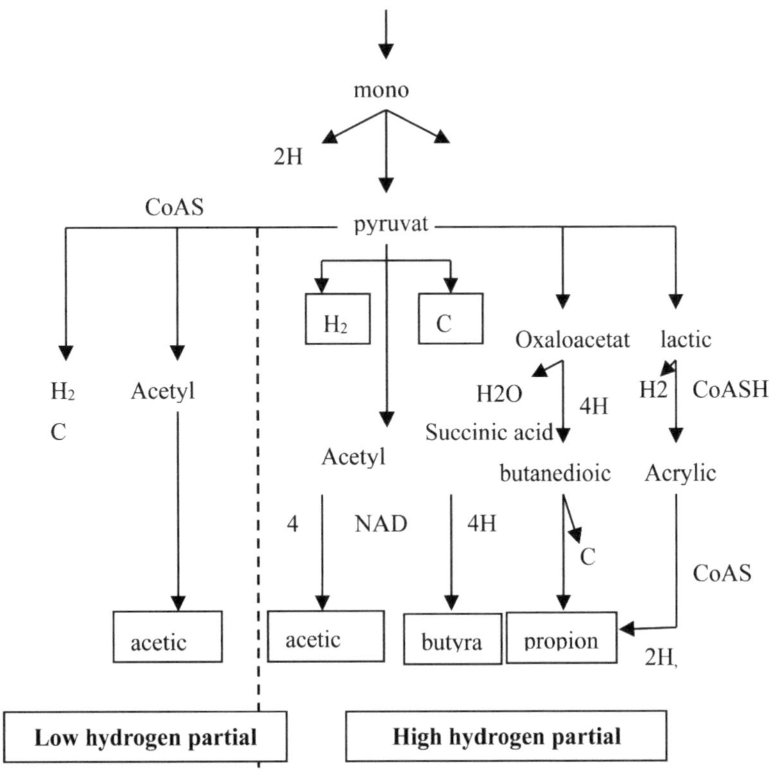

Figure 15.
Effect of hydrogen partial pressure on fermentation products.

	Fermentation reaction equation	Energy conversion rate (%)
(1)	$C_6H_{12}O_6 + 2H_2O—2CH_3COOH + 2CO_2 + 4H_2$	33.5
(2)	$4C_6H_{12}O_6—2CH_3COOH + 3CH_3CH_2CH_2COOH + 8CO_2 + 8H_2$	16.8
(3)	$C_6H_{12}O_6—3CH_4 + 3CO_2$	83.2
(4)	$C_6H_{12}O_6 + 2H_2O—2CH_4 + 4CO_2 + 4H_2$	89.9

Note: The energy conversion rate of hydrogen and methane production through joint fermentation is based on the ratio of the calorific value of methane and hydrogen to that of glucose (the calorific values of glucose, hydrogen, and methane are 2888, 242, and 801 kJ/mol, respectively).

Table 10.
Energy conversion of different fermentation reactions using glucose as substrate.

metabolites, such as volatile fatty acid (VFA) and alcohols (acetate, butyrate, and ethanol). With glucose as substrate and acetic acid as the only intermediate metabolite, 1 mol of glucose has a maximum theoretical hydrogen production rate of 4 mol, which is called the Thauer Limit. However, in the actual fermentation process, the intermediate metabolite is often a mixture of acetate and butyrate. Even if the maximum theoretical value of hydrogen production can be achieved, there is obviously energy stored in intermediate metabolites, which are the best substrates for methanogens, and these metabolites can be used by methanogens to produce methane (**Table 10**).

Based on the calorific values of glucose, hydrogen, and methane, we can theoretically calculate the energy conversion efficiency of different anaerobic digestion reaction processes:

1. Glucose as the substrate, the ideal fermentation is acetic acid as the only intermediate metabolite. The system has a maximum hydrogen production of up to 4 mol, which is the Thauer Limit. At this time, the energy conversion efficiency of the reaction is 33.5%, indicating that the carbon and hydrogen sources in the substrate are still stored in the intermediate metabolites of acetic acid and have not been released.

2. The actual fermentation is that the intermediate metabolite is a mixture of acetate, butyrate, and ethanol, and even if the hydrogen production in the system can reach the maximum, the energy conversion efficiency of the reaction is the lowest, only 16.8%, indicating that the carbon source and hydrogen source in the substrate are still stored in the intermediate metabolite in large quantities, awaiting further digestion and degradation in the next step.

3. If the energy stored in intermediate metabolites is completely released to produce methane, that is, the mixture of acetate, butyrate, and ethanol continues to ferment and degrade to produce methane, the energy conversion rate of the reaction can reach a relatively high 83.2%. It is precisely these intermediate metabolites that become the best substrates for methanogens and are fully utilized by methanogens that can achieve better energy conversion effects.

4. The optimal situation is that the hydrogen generated in the metabolic process is collected in time, and accompanied by acetate, butyrate, ethanol, and other intermediate metabolites to further produce methane, in theory, the highest energy recovery efficiency can be obtained, that is, the energy recovery

efficiency of combined hydrogen and methane production is not only far greater than that of hydrogen production alone, but also greater than that of methane production in anaerobic digestion alone.

5.5 Conclusion

Due to the low energy values involved in anaerobic metabolism processes (approximately 15.5 kJ/mol), we can analyze from ATP energetics:

Under standard conditions, the synthesis of 1 mole of ATP (as the universal value of metabolic energy of cells) requires +32 kJ/mol; under normal cell growth environment ([ATP] = 10 mM, [ADP] = 1 mM, and [Pi] = 10 mM), +50 kJ/mol is required, including the heat loss of 20 kJ/mol during cell metabolism. A total of +70 kJ/mol is required. Because the hydrolysis of one molecule of ATP will have three protons passing through the membrane structure, which is equivalent to one-third of the energy value, the minimum metabolic reaction free energy value at the disposal of the microorganisms is −20 kJ/mol, which is the minimum energy requirement for the survival of the symbiotic flora.

The proposal of the typical syntrophic symbiosis in the 1960s and the H_2 hypothesis in the 1970s both support the view that different flora live together (although the energy value of the syntrophic flora is low):

1. A typical example of symbiosis in the 1960s

   Marvin P. Bryant from the University of Illinois in the United States proposed a mixed culture (*Methanobacillus omelianskii*), in which the two are in thermodynamic equilibrium and beneficial for their growth:

$$\text{S organism}: 2CH_3CH_2OH + 2H_2O \rightarrow 2CH_3COO^- + 4H_2 + 2H^+ \quad \Delta G^{O'} = +19\ \text{kJ} \quad (16)$$

$$\text{MoH strain}: 4H_2 + 3CO_2 \rightarrow CH_4 + 2H_2O \quad \Delta G^{O'} = -131\ \text{kJ/methane} \quad (17)$$

$$\text{Co}-\text{culture}: 2CH_3CH_2OH + CO_2 \rightarrow 2CH_3COO^- + 2H^+ + CH_4 \quad \Delta G^{O'} = -112\ \text{kJ/methane} \quad (18)$$

1. The H_2 hypothesis theory in the 1970s

   Assuming that the host (methanogenic archaea) cannot synthesize enough ATP, while the symbiote (releasing H_2, CO_2, and acetic acid) can produce a large amount of ATP and export it to the peripheral space. If both parties coexist, and the symbiotic organism obtains organic matter from the external environment as a metabolic substrate, producing H_2 and energy continuously to supply the host, allowing the host to complete autotrophic metabolism in an anaerobic environment, this win-win interest drives them to coexist together, explaining the origin of energy metabolism.

The joint hydrogen and methane production process linked by interspecific hydrogen transfer can theoretically achieve the highest energy recovery efficiency. The hydrogen produced in the metabolic process can be collected in time, and the intermediate metabolites, such as acetate, butyrate, ethanol, and so on, can be further anaerobically digested to produce methane. The energy recovery efficiency of the joint hydrogen and methane production is not only far greater than that of hydrogen production alone, but also greater than that of methane production by anaerobic digestion alone.

6. Metabolic mechanism model of producing hydrogen then methane in anaerobic digestion system

Based on the analysis of the material metabolism process, energy sharing coordination, bacterial interaggregation, and symbiosis of anaerobic digestion system, the metabolic mechanism model of producing hydrogen then methane in anaerobic digestion system is proposed, which can better degrade organic matter, better release system energy, and better shorten fermentation reaction cycle, and is an ideal metabolic flow pathway of anaerobic digestion:

1. Metabolic process of anaerobically digested substances: H_2, CO_2, and acetic acid are important intermediate metabolites in the process of anaerobic digestion to produce hydrogen and methane. Theoretically, 33% of methane production comes from H_2 (using hydrogen and carbon dioxide to produce methane), and the remaining 67% comes from acetic acid (acetic acid oxidation reaction), which is accompanied by the mutual coupling of hydrogen consumption and methane production. It is the key metabolic process of the whole anaerobic digestion to produce methane, which not only realizes the interspecific hydrogen transfer, but also makes hydrogen and methane production possible in the anaerobic digestion process.

2. The interaggregation and syntrophic mechanism of different populations of microorganisms: Acetic acid oxidation and hydrogen-consuming methanogenic bacteria are coupled with each other, causing hydrolytic bacteria and methanogenic archaea to form relatively compact aggregates that are difficult to separate. They share the chemical energy (−15.5 kJ/mol) required for the survival of the flora by digesting the organic matter that cannot be degraded by themselves, and maintain normal life metabolic activities.

3. Energy collaborative sharing principle of anaerobic digestion: ATP energetics provides a good explanation for the low energy value of anaerobic metabolism (20 kJ/mol is the minimum energy requirement for the survival of mutualistic bacterial communities). The mutualistic symbiosis in the 1960s and the H_2 hypothesis in the 1970s both support the view of mutualistic symbiosis among different species. Symbiotic organisms obtain substrates from the external environment, and the energy (including H_2) produced by metabolism enables anaerobic hosts (methanogens) to achieve autotrophic metabolism. The energy interests of both parties drive them to coexist together, which is consistent with the origin of energy metabolism.

Author details

Fang Yin[1*], Junlin Ji[1,2] and Wudi Zhang[1]

1 School of Energy and Environment Science, Yunnan Normal University, Kunming, PR China

2 Economic Crop Technology Extension Station, Agricultural and Rural Bureau of Honghe Hani and Yi Autonomous Prefecture, Mengzi, China

*Address all correspondence to: yf6709@sina.com

References

[1] Elgarahy AM, Eloffy M, Hammad A, Saber AN, El-Sherif DM, Mohsen A, et al. Hydrogen production from wastewater, storage, economy, governance and applications: A review. Environmental Chemistry Letters. 2022; **20**:3453-3504. DOI: 10.1007/s10311-022-01480-3

[2] Ramprakash B, Lindblad P, Eaton-Rye JJ, Incharoensakdi A. Current strategies and future perspectives in biological hydrogen production: A review. Renewable and Sustainable Energy Reviews. 2022;**168**:112773. DOI: 10.1016/j.rser.2022.112773

[3] Holl E, Steinbrenner J, Merkle W, Krümpel J, Lansing S, Baier U, et al. Two-stage anaerobic digestion: State of technology and perspective roles in future energy systems. Bioresource Technology. 2022;**360**:127633. DOI: 10.1016/j.biortech.2022.127633

[4] Harirchi S, Wainaina S, Sar T, Nojoumi SA, Parchami M, Parchami M, et al. Microbiological insights into anaerobic digestion for biogas, hydrogen or volatile fatty acids (VFAs): A review. Bioengineered. 2022;**13**:6521-6557. DOI: 10.1080/21655979.2022.2035986

[5] Fang Y, Jue H, Wudi Z, Jianchang L, Rui X, Yubao C, et al. The study on co-fermentation of hydrogen and methane production by *Eupatorium adenophorum* spreng. Chinese Science Bulletin. 2010;**55**: 3469-3476. DOI: 10.1360/972009-1412

[6] Yunhua J, Wudi Z, Xiaohua Y, Linmao G. A experimental study on extended retention time of methane fermentation using eupatorium adenophrum Spreng. Journal of Yunnan University (Natural Sciences Edition). 1989;**11**:51-55. CNKI:SUN:YNDZ.0.1989-01-015

[7] Singh L, Wahid ZA. Methods for enhancing bio-hydrogen production from biological process: A review. Journal of Industrial and Engineering Chemistry. 2015;**21**:70-80. DOI: 10.1016/j.jiec.2014.05.035

[8] Woese CR. Archabacteria. Vol. 8. Netherlands: Elsevier; 2012

[9] Beaty PS, McInerncy MJ. Effects of organic acid anions on the growth and metabolism of Syntrophomonas wolfei in pure culture and in defined consortia. Applied and Environmental Microbiology. 1989;**55**:977-983. DOI: 10.1128/aem.55.4.977-983.1989

[10] Schauer NL, Ferry JG. Metabolism of formate in *Methanobacterium formicicum*. Journal of Bacteriology. 1980;**142**:800-807. DOI: 10.1128/jb.142.3.800-807.1980

[11] Daniels L, Sparling R, Sprott GD. The bioenergetics of methanogenesis. Biochimica et Biophysica Acta (BBA)-Reviews on Bioenergetics. 1984;**768**:113-163. DOI: 10.1016/0304-4173(84)90002-8

[12] Widdel F. Growth of methanogenic bacteria in pure culture with 2-propanol and other alcohols as hydrogen donors. Applied and Environmental Microbiology. 1986;**51**:1056-1062. DOI: 10.1128/aem.51.5.1056-1062.1986

[13] Zellner G, Winter J. Secondary alcohols as hydrogen donors for CO_2-reduction by methanogens. FEMS Microbiology Letters. 1987;**44**:323-328. DOI: 10.1111/j.1574-6968.1987.tb02309.x

[14] Patel GB, SPROTT GD. *Methanosaeta concilii* gen. nov., sp. nov. (“Methanothrix concilii”) and

Methanosaeta thermoacetophila nom. rev., comb. nov. International Journal of Systematic and Evolutionary Microbiology. 1990;**40**:79-82. DOI: 10.1099/00207713-40-1-79

[15] Oremland RS, Marsh LM, Polcin S. Methane production and simultaneous sulphate reduction in anoxic, salt marsh sediments. Nature. 1982;**296**:143-145. DOI: 10.1038/296143a0

[16] Danson MJ. Central metabolism of the Archaea. New Comprehensive Biochemistry. 1993;**26**:1-24. DOI: 10.1016/S0167-7306(08)60250-1

[17] Ferry JG. Methane from acetate. Journal of Bacteriology. 1992;**174**:5489-5495. DOI: 10.1128/jb.174.17.5489-5495.1992

[18] Barker HA. On the biochemistry of the methane fermentation. Archiv für Mikrobiologie. 1936;**7**:404-419. DOI: 10.1007/BF00407413

[19] Hattori S. Syntrophic acetate-oxidizing microbes in methanogenic environments. Microbes and Environments. 2008;**23**:118-127. DOI: 10.1264/jsme2.23.118

[20] Lee MJ, Zinder SH. Hydrogen partial pressures in a thermophilic acetate-oxidizing methanogenic coculture. Applied and Environmental Microbiology. 1988;**54**:1457-1461. DOI: 10.1128/aem.54.6.1457-1461.1988

[21] Zhang X, Wang Y, Jiao P, Zhang M, Deng Y, Jiang C, et al. Microbiome-functionality in anaerobic digesters: A critical review. Water Research. 2023; **249**:120891. DOI: 10.1016/j.watres.2023.120891

[22] Stams AJ, Plugge CM. Electron transfer in syntrophic communities of anaerobic bacteria and archaea. Nature Reviews. Microbiology. 2009;**7**:568-577. DOI: 10.1038/nrmicro2166

[23] Falkowski PG, Fenchel T, Delong EF. The microbial engines that drive Earth's biogeochemical cycles. Science. 2008; **320**:1034-1039. DOI: 10.1126/science.1153213

[24] Yang M, Watson J, Wang Z, Si B, Jiang W, Zhou B, et al. Understanding and design of two-stage fermentation: A perspective of interspecies electron transfer. Renewable and Sustainable Energy Reviews. 2022;**168**:112891. DOI: 10.1016/j.rser.2022.112891

[25] Thiele JH, Zeikus JG. Control of interspecies electron flow during anaerobic digestion: Significance of formate transfer versus hydrogen transfer during syntrophic methanogenesis in flocs. Applied and Environmental Microbiology. 1988;**54**: 20-29. DOI: 10.1128/aem.54.1.20-29.1988

[26] Tilche A, Galatola M. The potential of bio-methane as bio-fuel/bio-energy for reducing greenhouse gas emissions: A qualitative assessment for Europe in a life cycle perspective. Water Science and Technology. 2008;**57**:1683-1692. DOI: 10.2166/wst.2008.039

[27] Stams AJ, De Bok FA, Plugge CM, Van Eekert MH, Dolfing J, Schraa G. Exocellular electron transfer in anaerobic microbial communities. Environmental Microbiology. 2006;**8**: 371-382. DOI: 10.1111/j.1462-2920.2006.00989.x

[28] Sharma P, Bano A, Singh SP, Srivastava SK, Singh SP, Iqbal HM, et al. Different stages of microbial community during the anaerobic digestion of food waste. Journal of Food Science and Technology. 2023;**60**:2079-2091. DOI: 10.1007/s13197-022-05477-2

[29] Su K, Li L, Wang Q, Cao R. A review on the interspecies electron transfer of methane production in anaerobic digestion system. Fermentation. 2023;**9**: 467. DOI: 10.3390/fermentation9050467

[30] Schink B. Energetics of syntrophic cooperation in methanogenic degradation. Microbiology and Molecular Biology Reviews. 1997;**61**(2): 262-280. DOI: 10.1128/mmbr.61.2.262-280.1997

[31] Barker HA. Studies upon the methane-producing bacteria. Archiv für Mikrobiologie. 1936;7:420-438. DOI: 10.1007/BF00407414

[32] Thauer RK, Kaster A-K, Seedorf H, Buckel W, Hedderich R. Methanogenic archaea: Ecologically relevant differences in energy conservation. Nature Reviews. Microbiology. 2008;**6**: 579-591. DOI: 10.1038/nrmicro1931

[33] Iannotti E, Kafkewitz D, Wolin M, Bryant M. Glucose fermentation products of *Ruminococcus albus* grown in continuous culture with *Vibrio succinogenes*: Changes caused by interspecies transfer of H2. Journal of Bacteriology. 1973;**114**:1231-1240

[34] Müller N, Griffin BM, Stingl U, Schink B. Dominant sugar utilizers in sediment of Lake Constance depend on syntrophic cooperation with methanogenic partner organisms. Environmental Microbiology. 2008;**10**: 1501-1511. DOI: 10.1111/j.1462-2920.2007.01565.x

[35] Barker H. Studies upon the methane fermentation. IV. The isolation and culture of *Methanobacterium omelianskii*. Antonie Van Leeuwenhoek. 1939;**6**:201-220. DOI: 10.1007/BF02146187

[36] Brill WJ, Wolfe R. Acetaldehyde oxidation by methanobacillus–A new ferredoxin-dependent reaction. Nature. 1966;**212**:253-255. DOI: 10.1038/212253a0

[37] Bryant M, Wolin E, Wolin M, Wolfe R. *Methanobacillus omelianskii*, a symbiotic association of two species of bacteria. Archiv für Mikrobiologie. 1967; **59**:20-31. DOI: 10.1007/BF00406313

[38] Gray MW, Doolittle WF. Has the endosymbiont hypothesis been proven? Microbiological Reviews. 1982;**46**:1-42. DOI: 10.1128/mr.46.1.1-42.1982

[39] Mand TD, Metcalf WW. Energy conservation and hydrogenase function in methanogenic archaea, in particular the genus Methanosarcina. Microbiology and Molecular Biology Reviews. 2019;**83**: 1-22. DOI: 10.1128/MMBR.00020-19

[40] Zabranska J, Pokorna D. Bioconversion of carbon dioxide to methane using hydrogen and hydrogenotrophic methanogens. Biotechnology Advances. 2018;**36**:707-720. DOI: 10.1016/j.biotechadv.2017.12.003

[41] Basile A, Campanaro S, Kovalovszki A, Zampieri G, Rossi A, Angelidaki I, et al. Revealing metabolic mechanisms of interaction in the anaerobic digestion microbiome by flux balance analysis. Metabolic Engineering. 2020;**62**:138-149. DOI: 10.1016/j.ymben.2020.08.013

[42] Embley TM, Finlay BJ, Dyal PL, Hirt RP, Wilkinson M, Williams A. Multiple origins of anaerobic ciliates with hydrogenosomes within the radiation of aerobic ciliates. Proceedings of the Royal Society of London - Series B: Biological Sciences. 1995;**262**:87-93. DOI: 10.1098/rspb.1995.0180

[43] Beh M, Strauss G, Huber R, Stetter K-O, Fuchs G. Enzymes of the reductive citric acid cycle in the autotrophic

eubacterium *Aquifex pyrophilus* and in the archaebacterium *Thermoproteus neutrophilus*. Archives of Microbiology. 1993;**160**:306-311. DOI: 10.1007/BF00292082

[44] Fuchs G. CO_2 fixation in acetogenic bacteria: Variations on a theme. FEMS Microbiology Reviews. 1986;**2**:181-213. DOI: 10.1111/j.1574-6968.1986.tb01859.x

[45] Nakanishi-Matsui M, Futai M. Stochastic rotational catalysis of proton pumping F-ATPase. Philosophical Transactions of the Royal Society B: Biological Sciences. 2008;**363**:2135-2142. DOI: 10.1098/rstb.2008.2266

[46] Kosaka T, Kato S, Shimoyama T, Ishii S, Abe T, Watanabe K. The genome of *Pelotomaculum thermopropionicum* reveals niche-associated evolution in anaerobic microbiota. Genome Research. 2008;**18**:442-448. DOI: 10.1101/gr.7136508

[47] McInerney MJ, Bryant MP, Pfennig N. Anaerobic bacterium that degrades fatty acids in syntrophic association with methanogens. Archives of Microbiology. 1979;**122**:129-135. DOI: 10.1007/BF00411351

[48] Diekert G. CO_2 reduction to acetate in anaerobic bacteria. FEMS Microbiology Reviews. 1990;**7**:391-395. DOI: 10.1111/j.1574-6968.1990.tb04942.x

[49] Piché-Choquette S, Constant P. Molecular hydrogen, a neglected key driver of soil biogeochemical processes. Applied and Environmental Microbiology. 2019;**85**:e02418-e02418. DOI: 10.1128/AEM.02418-18

[50] Kumar K, Anand A, Moholkar VS. Molecular Hydrogen (H2) Metabolism in Microbes: A Special Focus on Biohydrogen Production. Biohydrogen-Advances and Processes. Germany: Springer; 2024. pp. 25-58

[51] Carepo M, Baptista J, Pamplona A, Fauque G, Moura J, Reis M. Hydrogen metabolism in *Desulfovibrio desulfuricans* strain New Jersey (NCIMB 8313)—Comparative study with D. Vulgaris and D. Gigas species. Anaerobe. 2002;**8**:325-332. DOI: 10.1016/S1075-9964(03)00007-6

[52] Sawers R. Formate and its Role in Hydrogen Production in Escherichia Coli. England: Portland Press Ltd.; 2005

[53] McInerney MJ, Struchtemeyer CG, Sieber J, Mouttaki H, Stams AJ, Schink B, et al. Physiology, ecology, phylogeny, and genomics of microorganisms capable of syntrophic metabolism. Annals of the New York Academy of Sciences. 2008;**1125**:58-72. DOI: 10.1196/annals.1419.005

[54] Schmidt JE, Ahring BK. Interspecies electron transfer during propionate and butyrate degradation in mesophilic, granular sludge. Applied and Environmental Microbiology. 1995;**61**:2765-2767. DOI: 10.1128/aem.61.7.2765-2767.1995

[55] Lettinga G, Zehnder A, Grotenhuis J, Hulshoff Pol L. Granular Anaerobic Sludge; Microbiology and Technology. Wageningen, The Netherlands: Centre for Agricultural Publishing and Documentation (PUDOC), Wageningen; 1988

[56] Tomlinson GA, Koch TK, Hochstein L. The metabolism of carbohydrates by extremely halophilic bacteria: Glucose metabolism via a modified Entner-Doudoroff pathway. Canadian Journal of Microbiology. 1974;**20**:1085-1091. DOI: 10.1139/m74-170

[57] Kates M, Kushner DJ, Matheson A. The Biochemistry of Archaea

(Archaebacteria). Netherlands: Elsevier; 1993

[58] Bin Y, Fang Y, Jing L, Xingling Z, Shiqing L, Ling X, et al. Energy efficiency of hydrogen and methane coupled production by cow dung fermentation. China Biogas. 2014;**32**:53-56. DOI: 10.3969/j.issn.1000-1166.2014.01.011

[59] Zhihong W, Shouhua L. Study on energy conversion efficiency of biogas fermentation. Journal of Liaoning Teachers College. 2002;**4**:84-87. DOI: 10.3969/j.issn.1008-5688.2002.03.030

[60] Cheng J, Xie B, Zhou J, Song W, Cen K. Cogeneration of H_2 and CH_4 from water hyacinth by two-step anaerobic fermentation. International Journal of Hydrogen Energy. 2010;**35**:3029-3035. DOI: 10.1016/j.ijhydene.2009.07.012

[61] Castelló E, Ferraz-Junior ADN, Andreani C, del Pilar A-RM, Borzacconi L, Buitrón G, et al. Stability problems in the hydrogen production by dark fermentation: Possible causes and solutions. Renewable and Sustainable Energy Reviews. 2020;**119**:109602. DOI: 10.1016/j.rser.2019.109602

[62] Xie B, Cheng J, Zhou J, Song W, Liu J, Cen K. Production of hydrogen and methane from potatoes by two-phase anaerobic fermentation. Bioresource Technology. 2008;**99**:5942-5946. DOI: 10.1016/j.biortech.2007.10.048

[63] Hallenbeck P. Fundamentals of the fermentative production of hydrogen. Water Science and Technology. 2005;**52**: 21-29. DOI: 10.2166/wst.2005.0494

[64] Hallenbeck PC, Benemann JR. Biological hydrogen production; fundamentals and limiting processes. International Journal of Hydrogen Energy. 2002;**27**:1185-1193. DOI: 10.1016/S0360-3199(02)00131-3

Chapter 5

The Hidden Influence of Methanogens in the Gut Microbiota

Özge Dua Zengin and Sevcan Aydin

Abstract

Methanogens are a distinct group of archaea characterized by their ability to produce methane as a metabolic byproduct. These microorganisms play a crucial role in the gut microbiota, influencing various physiological processes, including digestion, immune modulation, and the gut-brain axis. Although their abundance is lower compared to bacteria, the impact of methanogens on health and disease is significant. This review aims to elucidate the hidden influence of methanogens within the gut microbiota, with a particular focus on their associations with gastrointestinal and neurological disorders. By synthesizing recent findings, the review seeks to underscore the critical role of methanogens in health and disease and to offer novel insights into potential therapeutic strategies aimed at targeting these archaea.

Keywords: methanogens, archaea, human archaeome, gut microbiota, gastrointestinal health

1. Introduction

The human gastrointestinal microbiota, a complex and dynamic ecosystem, is home to a vast array of microorganisms, including bacteria, viruses, fungi, and archaea [1]. While much of the research has focused on bacteria, recent advances have brought attention to another, often overlooked domain of life: the archaea, in human health and disease. The human archaeome, which refers to the collection of archaeal species within the human body, is increasingly understood to play a significant role in maintaining health and contributing to disease [2]. Unlike bacteria, archaea are a distinct domain of life characterized by unique molecular structures, metabolic pathways, and ecological roles [3]. Although their presence in the human microbiome is less abundant than bacteria, their impact is profound, particularly in terms of metabolic processes and interactions with the immune system [4].

Archaea are distinct from bacteria and eukaryotes in terms of their cellular structure and metabolic pathways [3]. Methanogens, a specialized group of archaea, are especially prevalent in the human gut, where they play a vital role in the final stages of anaerobic digestion [5]. Species such as *Methanobrevibacter smithii* and *Methanosphaera stadtmanae* are key players in this process, converting hydrogen and carbon dioxide into methane. This methanogenesis process is essential for maintaining hydrogen balance in the gut, which, in turn, supports the efficient fermentation of dietary fibers by bacteria [6]. The end products of this fermentation, particularly short-chain fatty acids (SCFAs) like acetate, propionate, and butyrate, are crucial for host health [5]. SCFAs serve as a primary energy source for colonocytes, support the maintenance of gut barrier integrity, and exert anti-inflammatory effects that are vital for immune homeostasis [7]. Methanogens are particularly associated with the modulation of the gut-brain axis, a bidirectional communication network that connects the central nervous system (CNS) with the gastrointestinal system [8]. Disruptions in this axis have been associated with a range of neurological disorders, including anxiety, depression, and neurodegenerative diseases. Methanogens may influence these conditions by affecting gut motility, immune responses, and the production of neurotransmitters [2].

In addition to their role in the gut, archaea are also present in other body sites, contributing to different physiological processes. For example, ammonia-oxidizing archaea (AOA) are found on the skin and in the upper aerodigestive tract (UAT), where they are involved in the oxidation of ammonia to nitrite. This process is crucial for regulating skin pH, which can influence skin conditions such as acne, and for maintaining respiratory health. The presence of archaea in these diverse environments underscores their adaptability and ecological versatility within the human body. For instance, methanogens in the gut have been associated with gastrointestinal disorders such as irritable bowel syndrome (IBS) disease, obesity and allergic diseases. In the skin and UAT, shifts in archaeal populations have been observed in conditions like refractory sinusitis and vaginosis [2]. Moreover, recent research has highlighted the complex interactions between archaea and the human immune system. Certain archaeal molecules, such as RNA and unique glycerolipids, can trigger immune responses by activating specific receptors, including Toll-like receptor 8 (TLR8) and C-type lectin receptors like MINCLE [9]. These interactions suggest that while archaea are not direct pathogens, they can influence immune function and potentially contribute to inflammatory processes [10].

This review explores the hidden influence of methanogens within the gut microbiota, focusing on their connections to gastrointestinal and neurological disorders. By examining recent studies and integrating insights from multiple disciplines, we aim to provide a comprehensive understanding of how these archaea contribute to health and disease. The potential for targeting methanogens in therapeutic interventions will also be discussed, highlighting the need for continued research into this often-overlooked component of the human microbiome.

2. Methanogens in the human gut: Composition and function

Methanogens are a specialized group of archaea characterized by their ability to produce methane, a process that occurs under anaerobic conditions in the human gut [11]. These microorganisms are found in various environments, including wetlands, sediments, and the digestive tracts of ruminants, but they also play a crucial role in the human gastrointestinal system [10]. The human gut harbors a relatively small population of methanogens compared to bacteria, yet their metabolic activity has a disproportionate impact on gut physiology and microbial ecology.

The human gut hosts a diverse population of methanogens, with *M. smithii* being the most prevalent species, followed by *M. stadtmanae* and *Methanomassiliicoccus luminyensis*. Studies indicate that *M. smithii* and *M. stadtmanae* are the most dominant methanogens in the human gut microbiota, with prevalence rates reaching up to 95.7% for *M. smithii*. This high prevalence highlights their significant role in the gut ecosystem [12]. These organisms play a pivotal role in the anaerobic digestion process, where they facilitate the breakdown of complex carbohydrates into SCFAs, which are vital for maintaining gut health. Methanogenesis, the process by which methane is produced, has significant implications for gut health [6]. Methane is a non-toxic gas that is typically excreted in the breath or passed as flatulence. However, the production of methane is associated with slower intestinal transit times, a factor that can contribute to gastrointestinal disorders such as constipation-predominant IBS (IBS-C) [13]. Studies have shown that individuals who are methane-positive, as determined by breath testing, often experience delayed colonic transit compared to methane-negative individuals [14]. This suggests that methanogens, by producing methane, play a direct role in regulating gut motility.

Beyond their role in gut motility, methanogens also influence the overall composition and function of the gut microbiota [15]. The presence of methanogens can impact the balance of other microbial populations, particularly those involved in the production of SCFAs, which are important for maintaining gut barrier integrity, modulating inflammation, and providing energy to colonocytes [7]. Methanogens rely on syntrophic interactions with other gut bacteria that produce substrates necessary for methanogenesis. These interactions are crucial for efficient metabolic regulation and are key to the stability and resilience of the gut microbiome [12]. Methanogens' ability to modulate hydrogen levels ensures that bacterial fermentation processes remain efficient, leading to a stable and resilient gut microbiome [16]. The composition and activity of methanogens in the human gut are influenced by various factors, including diet, age, and genetics [15]. Diets rich in fiber, for example, promote the growth of hydrogen-producing bacteria, which in turn support methanogen activity. Conversely, diets low in fermentable substrates may reduce the availability of hydrogen, potentially leading to lower methanogen populations [16]. Understanding these interactions is crucial for developing dietary interventions aimed at modulating methanogen activity to improve gut health (**Figure 1**).

Recent research compared the results of the lactulose breath test (LBT) between patients with irritable bowel syndrome and healthy individuals. The findings indicated that LBT was unable to distinguish between IBS patients and healthy subjects. Additionally, methane production in IBS patients was linked to constipation, while it was inversely related to diarrhea. The study highlights that the current LBT criteria are not effective for diagnosing IBS [17].

The diversity of methanogens in the human gut is not limited to *M. smithii* and the other methanogens already mentioned. Other methanogens, such as *Methanobacterium formicicum* and *Methanobrevibacter ruminantium*, have also been detected, though less commonly. These species, while not as well-characterized as *M. smithii*, contribute to the overall metabolic activity of the gut microbiota and highlight the potential for a broader range of methanogens to influence gut health [18]. As research continues to explore the human archaeome, it is becoming increasingly clear that methanogens play a multifaceted role in the gut. Their ability to interact with other microbial species, influence gut motility, and impact overall microbial balance underscores their importance in maintaining gut health and homeostasis. By deepening our understanding of these interactions, we can better appreciate the contributions of methanogens to both health and disease.

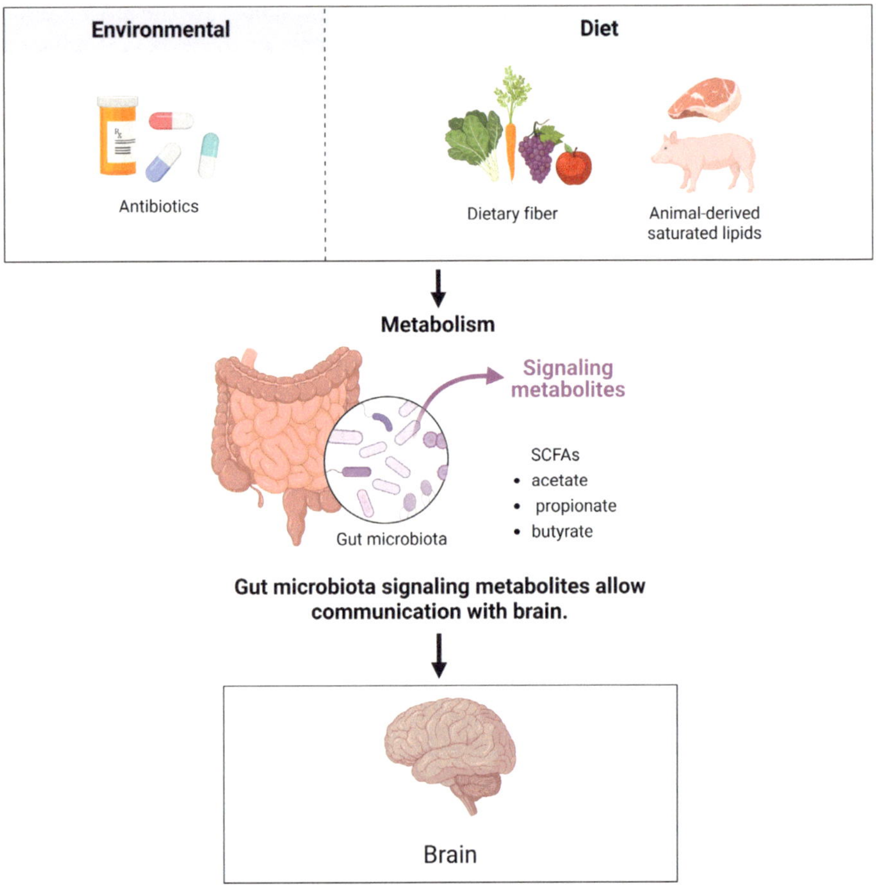

Figure 1.
Environmental and dietary factors influencing gut microbiota metabolism and brain communication. Antibiotics and dietary components such as dietary fiber and animal-derived saturated lipids modulate gut microbiota composition and activity. This results in the production of short-chain fatty acids (SCFAs) like acetate, propionate, and butyrate. These signaling metabolites enable the gut microbiota to communicate with the brain, highlighting the interplay between gut health and neurological function. (Created in BioRender.com).

3. Methane production and gastrointestinal disorders

Methanogens have been implicated in various gastrointestinal disorders, with their activity linked to both beneficial and pathological outcomes. One of the most extensively studied associations is between methanogens and constipation-predominant irritable bowel syndrome. Methane production is known to slow down gastrointestinal transit, which can worsen constipation symptoms. Elevated levels of methane are linked to reduced gut motility, further intensifying the discomfort associated with constipation. Research indicates that methane can impact motor functions within the gastrointestinal tract, occasionally increasing intestinal contractions. This relationship is especially significant for individuals with constipation-predominant irritable bowel syndrome, as they often exhibit higher methane levels, which are correlated with more pronounced constipation symptoms [19].

Clinical studies have consistently demonstrated that patients with IBS-C have elevated levels of breath methane, reflecting increased methanogen activity in the gut. Methane production correlates with delayed intestinal transit times, which exacerbate the symptoms of IBS-C, including abdominal discomfort, bloating, and constipation [20].

The pathophysiology of IBS-C in the context of methanogen activity involves the modulation of smooth muscle contractions within the gastrointestinal tract. Methane is believed to influence the enteric nervous system, altering the release of neurotransmitters that regulate peristalsis [21]. For instance, methane may reduce the activity of serotonin, a neurotransmitter critical for promoting gut motility. This reduction in serotonin activity could explain the prolonged transit times observed in methane-positive patients with IBS-C. Moreover, the presence of methanogens, particularly *M. smithii*, has been associated with an altered gut microbiota composition, which may further contribute to the dysbiosis observed in IBS patients [22].

In addition to IBS-C, methanogens are also implicated in small intestinal bacterial overgrowth (SIBO), a condition characterized by an excessive proliferation of bacteria in the small intestine [23]. In clinical practice, the lactulose breath test is widely used to assess small intestinal bacterial overgrowth and other gastrointestinal conditions, including IBS. Lactulose, a non-absorbable sugar, is ingested and metabolized by gut bacteria, producing hydrogen and methane, which can be measured in exhaled breath. The test typically involves administering a standard dose of lactulose (10 g), followed by breath sampling at 15–20-minute intervals for up to 3 hours. The key principle behind the LBT is the identification of abnormal gas production profiles. A normal result shows a single peak of hydrogen or methane when lactulose reaches the colon. In contrast, individuals with SIBO may exhibit an early peak when lactulose is metabolized by bacteria in the small intestine, followed by the normal peak upon entry into the colon [23].

Studies have demonstrated that while hydrogen breath tests alone can miss cases, particularly those involving methane-producing archaea, simultaneous measurement of both hydrogen and methane offers improved diagnostic accuracy. Approximately 30–50% of IBS patients may produce methane, which has been linked to constipation-predominant IBS due to methane's effect of slowing intestinal transit. Recent advancements have made dual detection more accessible, contributing to better clinical management of IBS and SIBO [23].

Methane-positive SIBO, also referred to as intestinal methanogen overgrowth (IMO), is distinguished by its association with constipation rather than diarrhea, which is more common in hydrogen-dominant SIBO [24]. The presence of methanogens in the small intestine exacerbates symptoms by further slowing intestinal transit, leading to increased bacterial fermentation, gas production, and discomfort [25].

A recent study specifically examined the role of serotonin in IBS patients who produce methane (CH_4). Findings suggest that methane production may be linked to reduced serotonin levels in the gut, a neurotransmitter crucial for regulating intestinal motility. Lower serotonin levels can contribute to delayed transit times, offering a possible explanation for how methane impacts gastrointestinal function. In methane-producing IBS patients, serotonin levels were found to be lower than in those who only produce hydrogen, highlighting methane's potential influence on gut motility dynamics [26].

The role of methanogens in other gastrointestinal disorders, such as inflammatory bowel disease (IBD) and colorectal cancer, is also of interest. In IBD, the contribution of methanogens to disease pathology remains unclear. However, some studies suggest that methanogen-related dysbiosis may influence the chronic inflammation characteristic of the disease [27]. In colorectal cancer, methanogens may impact tumorigenesis through their interactions with the gut microbiota and the immune system [28].

For instance, the production of methane and other metabolites by methanogens could create a microenvironment conducive to cancer progression [29]. According to Armougom et al. 2009, it has been determined that the concentration of *Lactobacillus* species increases in obese individuals, while the level of *M. smithii* rises in patients with anorexia nervosa. The study examined the bacterial communities in the feces of 20 obese patients, 9 patients with anorexia nervosa, and 20 normal-weight healthy controls. The results showed that the proportion of *Bacteroidetes* was reduced in the feces of obese individuals, while the *Lactobacillus* species were found at higher levels in obese patients. In patients with anorexia, the concentration of *M. smithii* was found to be significantly higher compared to the normal-weight control group [30]. These associations underscore the need for further research to elucidate the complex role of methanogens in gastrointestinal health and disease.

4. Methanogens and the gut-brain axis: Connections to neurological disorders

The gut-brain axis is a sophisticated communication network that connects the central nervous system with the gastrointestinal system [31]. This bidirectional system comprises various pathways, including neural, hormonal, and immunological mechanisms, enabling the gut and brain to affect each other's functions [32]. Recent research has highlighted the significant role of the gut microbiota in modulating the gut-brain axis, with disruptions in this axis linked to a variety of neurological and psychiatric disorders [33]. Methanogens, as key members of the gut microbiota, are emerging as important players in this intricate network [34].

One of the key mechanisms by which methanogens may influence neurological health is through their impact on neurotransmitter production. The gut microbiota is essential for the synthesis and metabolism of neurotransmitters, including serotonin, dopamine, and gamma-aminobutyric acid (GABA). Methanogens, by modulating the activity of other microbes in the gut, can affect the levels of these neurotransmitters [16]. For example, reduced microbial diversity, which is often associated with high methanogen levels, can lead to imbalances in the production of short-chain fatty acids, which have neuroactive properties. SCFAs can cross the blood-brain barrier and influence brain function, potentially contributing to the development or exacerbation of neurological conditions [15]. A recent study revealed the presence of methanogens, specifically *Methanobrevibacter oralis*, in brain abscess samples, suggesting that methanogens may play a role in central nervous system infections. The findings indicated that *M. oralis* could be neurotoxic, with its methane production having potential negative effects on neural tissue [35].

A recent study revealed that Bacteroides and other gut bacteria are capable of producing GABA, with these pathways actively expressed in healthy individuals. Additionally, a negative correlation was observed between the relative abundance of Bacteroides and brain signatures linked to neurological disorders such as depression. The research also suggests that methanogens may play a role in GABA production within the gut, highlighting its potential significance in the pathogenesis of neurological disorders [36].

The relationship between methanogens and the gut-brain axis extends beyond gut motility. Methane production by *M. oralis* may act as a neurotoxin, as demonstrated in experimental studies where it caused increased mortality in neural tissue models [35]. Methane has been shown to exert anti-inflammatory effects, which may influence systemic inflammation-a key factor in the development of neurodegenerative diseases such as Alzheimer's and Parkinson's. Chronic low-grade inflammation, often associated with gut dysbiosis, can contribute to the pathogenesis of these conditions by promoting neuroinflammation and oxidative stress. By modulating inflammation, methanogens may have a protective role in maintaining brain health [15]. Recent studies have also explored the potential link between methanogens and mood disorders. Patients with IBS, particularly those with IBS-C, often exhibit comorbid conditions such as anxiety and depression. The altered gut motility and inflammation associated with methane production may contribute to these psychological symptoms. For example, a study by Wang et al. found that patients with IBS-C who were methane-positive had higher levels of anxiety and depression compared to methane-negative patients. This suggests that methanogens, by influencing the gut-brain axis, may play a role in the development or exacerbation of mood disorders [37].

In addition to mood disorders, the gut-brain axis is implicated in the pathophysiology of autism spectrum disorder (ASD). Alterations in the gut microbiota have been observed in individuals with ASD, including changes in the abundance of methanogens. Some studies have suggested that the presence of methanogens may be linked to gastrointestinal symptoms commonly seen in ASD, such as constipation [38]. These findings raise the possibility that methanogens could contribute to the gut-brain interactions that influence the behavioral and cognitive features of ASD.

The potential for targeting methanogens to modulate the gut-brain axis presents new therapeutic opportunities. Interventions aimed at reducing methane production, such as antibiotics or dietary modifications, could help alleviate symptoms associated with both gastrointestinal and neurological disorders [20]. Additionally, psychobiotics—probiotics that influence mental health—may offer a novel approach to treating conditions like anxiety and depression by modulating methanogen activity and restoring balance to the gut microbiota [39]. Overall, methanogens play a significant role in the gut-brain axis, influencing both gastrointestinal and neurological health. By understanding the mechanisms through which methanogens affect this communication network, we can develop targeted therapies that address the underlying causes of intestinal-brain disorders and improve patient outcomes.

5. Methanogens and immune modulation

Methanogens interact with the human immune system in complex and multifaceted ways, influencing both innate and adaptive immunity. These archaea can activate various immune cells, including dendritic cells, macrophages, and T cells, through mechanisms that are still being uncovered. One key pathway involves the recognition of microbe-associated molecular patterns (MAMPs) by Toll-like receptors (TLRs), particularly TLR7 and TLR8, which detect single-stranded RNA-a feature common to methanogens. The activation of these TLRs triggers downstream signaling cascades that result in the production of proinflammatory cytokines such as IL-1β, IL-6, and TNF-α [40]. These cytokines play critical roles in orchestrating the immune response, driving inflammation, and recruiting other immune cells to sites of infection or injury (**Figure 2**).

The activation of the NLRP3 inflammasome by methanogens is particularly relevant in the context of allergic and atopic diseases. The NLRP3 inflammasome is a multiprotein complex that plays a central role in the maturation and secretion of IL-1β, a cytokine that is pivotal in the initiation of inflammatory responses.

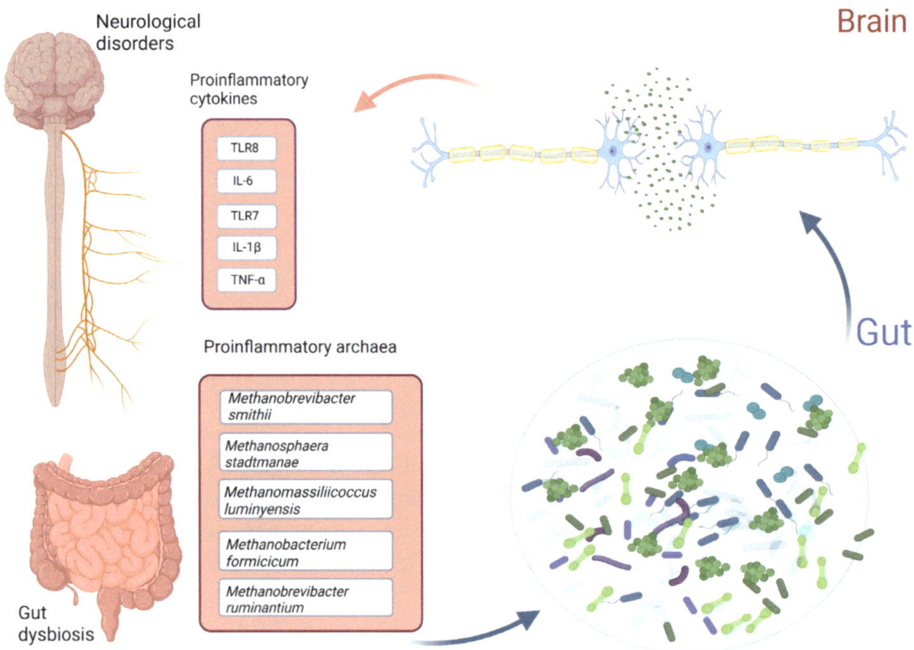

Figure 2.
This figure illustrates the role of methanogenic archaea in the gut-brain axis and their potential impact on neurological disorders. Gut dysbiosis can lead to the proliferation of proinflammatory archaea species. These archaea can stimulate an inflammatory response in the gut by producing proinflammatory molecules. This inflammatory response leads to the activation of Toll-like receptors (such as TLR7 and TLR8) and the release of proinflammatory cytokines, including IL-6, IL-1β, and TNF-α. These inflammatory signals can travel to the brain, potentially causing inflammation in neurons and contributing to neurological disorders. The image shows the pathway of inflammatory molecules from the gut to the brain, where they may disrupt neuronal function and compromise blood–brain barrier integrity, activating pathways associated with neurological conditions. (Created in BioRender.com).

In conditions such as asthma and allergic rhinitis, methanogen-induced activation of the NLRP3 inflammasome could exacerbate inflammation, contributing to the severity of these diseases. Additionally, methanogens have been implicated in the modulation of T helper cell responses, particularly the differentiation of Th1, Th2, and Th17 cells, which are central to the immune response in allergic conditions [16]. According to Choileáin et al., the relationship between T cells, which are part of the immune system, and the diversity of the gut microbiome in patients with multiple sclerosis (MS) was investigated. The study identified decreased levels of methanogens, such as *Methanobrevibacter*, in the gut microbiome of MS patients, suggesting potential effects on immune responses. Additionally, it was found that increased CXCR3+ T cells, particularly Th1 cells, were associated with reduced gut microbiome diversity, which may contribute to MS pathology [41].

In addition to their proinflammatory effects, methanogens may also exhibit immunoregulatory properties. The SCFAs produced by the fermentation of dietary fibers by gut bacteria, a process facilitated by methanogens, are known to promote the differentiation of regulatory T cells (Tregs). Tregs are essential for maintaining immune tolerance, preventing autoimmunity, and resolving inflammation. By supporting SCFA production, methanogens may indirectly contribute to the regulation of immune responses, highlighting their dual role in both promoting and resolving inflammation [42].

Based on recent research, methanoarchaea such as *M. stadtmanae* and *M. smithii* have been found to activate immune responses by increasing the expression of CD86 and CD197 on antigen-presenting cells. This leads to T cell-mediated immune responses. Such modulation of both innate and adaptive immune systems suggests a potential role for methanogens in inflammatory bowel diseases and highlights the importance of phagocytosis in immune cell activation [13].

Moreover, methanogens have been associated with the modulation of antimicrobial peptide production. These peptides are crucial for maintaining the integrity of mucosal surfaces and preventing the overgrowth of pathogenic microbes. The ability of methanogens to influence antimicrobial peptide production suggests that they play a role in maintaining the balance between commensal and pathogenic microorganisms, further emphasizing their importance in immune homeostasis [44].

6. Therapeutic potential of targeting methanogens

The clinical implications of methanogen activity in the human gut are broad, extending from gastrointestinal disorders to neurological conditions. As research continues to uncover the connections between methanogens and health, new therapeutic strategies are being developed to target these archaea and improve patient outcomes.

Therapeutic strategies targeting methanogens include the use of antibiotics, probiotics, prebiotics, and dietary interventions. Rifaximin, a non-systemic antibiotic, has shown promise in reducing methane production and improving symptoms in patients with IBS-C. Studies have demonstrated that rifaximin, particularly when combined with neomycin, can effectively reduce methanogen populations in the gut, leading to improved gut motility and symptom relief. However, the long-term effects of antibiotic treatment on the gut microbiota and the potential for antibiotic resistance remain concerns that need to be addressed in future research [45].

Probiotics and prebiotics offer an alternative approach to modulating methanogen activity. Probiotics containing hydrogen-consuming bacteria, such as *Lactobacillus* and *Bifidobacterium* species, could potentially compete with methanogens for hydrogen, thereby reducing methane production. Prebiotics, on the other hand, could be used to promote the growth of beneficial microbes that outcompete methanogens for substrates [46]. Prebiotic fibers, such as inulin, fructo-oligosaccharides (FOS), and galacto-oligosaccharides (GOS), are fermented by gut bacteria, leading to the production of short-chain fatty acids and gases such as hydrogen [15]. This hydrogen can then be utilized by methanogens to produce methane. The availability of hydrogen as a substrate is a key factor influencing methanogen activity. Therefore, prebiotics that increase hydrogen production may indirectly promote methanogenesis, potentially impacting gut motility and microbial balance. These dietary interventions may help manage methanogen-related disorders by altering the composition and function of the gut microbiota. Future research should aim to clarify the interactions between different types of prebiotics and methanogens, exploring how these interactions influence gut health and disease. Understanding the conditions under which prebiotics either enhance or inhibit methanogen activity will be crucial for developing effective dietary strategies that optimize gut function while minimizing adverse effects. Additionally, the exploration of novel prebiotics that specifically target methanogens without disrupting the broader gut microbiota could open new avenues for managing conditions associated with altered methane production [12].

In addition to gastrointestinal disorders, the potential for targeting methanogens in the treatment of neurological conditions is an exciting area of research. As discussed earlier, methanogens influence the gut-brain axis and may contribute to mood disorders, neurodegenerative diseases, and autism spectrum disorder [15]. Psychobiotics, a class of probiotics that affect mental health, represent a novel therapeutic approach for these conditions. By modulating methanogen activity and restoring balance to the gut microbiota, psychobiotics could help alleviate symptoms associated with both gastrointestinal and neurological disorders.

The development of targeted therapies for methanogens also extends to dietary interventions. Diet plays a crucial role in shaping the gut microbiota, and specific dietary patterns may influence methanogen activity. For example, diets high in fiber promote the growth of hydrogen-producing bacteria, which in turn support methanogenesis. Conversely, low-fiber diets may reduce the availability of hydrogen, potentially leading to lower methanogen populations [10]. Understanding the relationship between diet and methanogen activity is essential for developing dietary interventions that can modulate the gut microbiota and improve health outcomes.

The concept of "archaebiotics," which involves the administration of specific methanogenic archaea to modulate gut microbiota, is also gaining attention as a potential therapeutic strategy. By harnessing the natural metabolic capabilities of methanogens, archaebiotics could help restore microbial balance and reduce disease risk [47]. Understanding the complex interactions between methanogens, other gut microbes, and the host is essential for developing effective therapeutic strategies that target methanogen activity.

7. Conclusions

The investigation into the influence of methanogens within the gut microbiota has revealed their potential importance in both health and disease. While these archaea appear to play a crucial role in maintaining gut health, it is essential to acknowledge that their relationship with human health is complex and multifaceted. Emerging research suggests that targeting methanogens could lead to innovative approaches for managing gastrointestinal disorders and a range of other health issues, including metabolic and immune-related complications. However, it is critical to approach these findings with caution. The interaction between methanogens and other microbial communities, as well as their impact on host physiology, remains an area of active investigation.

Although methanogen research holds promise for developing new therapeutic strategies, it is important to recognize that the pathway to clinical applications may be long and require extensive validation. The exploration of personalized medicine, informed by individual genetic and microbial profiles, could indeed pave the way for tailored interventions. However, the integration of methanogen-targeted therapies into clinical practice will necessitate a thorough understanding of their roles and interactions within the broader microbial ecosystem.

In conclusion, while the potential of methanogens to influence health outcomes is significant, it is essential to maintain a balanced view that considers the complexities of microbial interactions and the need for further research. Advancements in our understanding of methanogens could undoubtedly contribute to the evolution of modern medicine, but a holistic approach will be vital in ensuring the effectiveness and safety of future therapeutic interventions.

Acknowledgements

The author acknowledges the use of ChatGPT for language editing in the chapter.

Author details

Özge Dua Zengin and Sevcan Aydin*
Division of Biotechnology, Biology Department, Faculty of Science, Istanbul University, Istanbul, Turkey

*Address all correspondence to: sevcan.aydin@istanbul.edu.tr

References

[1] Hoffmann C, Dollive S, Grunberg S, Chen J, Li H, Wu GD, et al. Archaea and Fungi of the Human Gut Microbiome: Correlations with Diet and Bacterial Residents. PLoS One. 17 Jun 2013;**8**(6):e0066019

[2] Kuehnast T, Kumpitsch C, Mohammadzadeh R, Weichhart T, Moissl-Eichinger C, Heine H. Exploring the human archaeome: Its relevance for health and disease, and its complex interplay with the human immune system. FEBS Journal (John Wiley and Sons Inc). 2024

[3] Eckburg PB, Lepp PW, Relman DA. Archaea and their potential role in human disease. Infection and Immunity (Washington, DC, USA: American Society for Microbiology). 2003;**71**(2):591-596

[4] Bang C, Schmitz RA. Archaea associated with human surfaces: Not to be underestimated. FEMS Microbiology Reviews (Oxford University Press). 2015;**39**:631-648

[5] Nkamga VD, Henrissat B, Drancourt M. Archaea: Essential inhabitants of the human digestive microbiota. Human Microbiome Journal (Elsevier Ltd). 2017;**3**:1-8

[6] Dridi B, Henry M, Richet H, Raoult D, Drancourt M. Age-related prevalence of Methanomassiliicoccus luminyensis in the human gut microbiome. APMIS. 2012;**120**(10):773-777. DOI: 10.1111/j.1600-0463.2012.02899.x

[7] Liu P, Wang Y, Yang G, Zhang Q, Meng L, Xin Y, et al. The role of short-chain fatty acids in intestinal barrier function, inflammation, oxidative stress, and colonic carcinogenesis. Pharmacological Research (Academic Press). 2021;**165**:105-115

[8] Silva YP, Bernardi A, Frozza RL. The Role of Short-Chain Fatty Acids From Gut Microbiota in Gut-Brain Communication. Frontiers in Endocrinology. Frontiers Media S.A. 2020;**11**:25-35

[9] Oka S, Watanabe M, Ito E, Takeyama A, Matsuoka T, Arichi N, et al. Archaeal glycerolipids are recognized by C-type lectin receptor mincle. Journal of the American Chemical Society (Washington, D.C., USA: American Chemical Society). 2023;**145**(18):8538-8547

[10] Mafra D, Ribeiro M, Fonseca L, Regis B, Cardozo LFMF, Fragoso dos Santos H, et al. Archaea from the gut microbiota of humans: Could be linked to chronic diseases? Anaerobe (Academic Press). 2022;**77**:102-110

[11] Guindo CO, Davoust B, Drancourt M, Grine G. Diversity of methanogens in animals' gut. Microorganisms. 2020;**9**(1):13. DOI: 10.3390/microorganisms9010013

[12] Djemai K, Drancourt M, Tidjani Alou M. Bacteria and Methanogens in the Human Microbiome: a Review of Syntrophic Interactions. Microbial Ecology (Springer). 2022;**83**:536-554

[13] Kunkel D, Basseri RJ, Makhani MD, Chong K, Chang C, Pimentel M. Methane on breath testing is associated with constipation: A systematic review and meta-analysis. Digestive Diseases and Sciences (New York, NY, USA: Springer). 2011;**56**(6):1612-1618

[14] Singh P, Lembo A. Emerging Role of the Gut Microbiome in Irritable Bowel

Syndrome. Gastroenterology Clinics of North America (W.B. Saunders). 2021;**50**:523-545

[15] You M, Chen N, Yang Y, Cheng L, He H, Cai Y, et al. The gut microbiota–brain axis in neurological disorders. MedComm (John Wiley and Sons Inc). 2024;**5**:12-25

[16] Sereme Y, Mezouar S, Grine G, Mege JL, Drancourt M, Corbeau P, et al. Methanogenic Archaea: Emerging Partners in the Field of Allergic Diseases. Clinical Reviews in Allergy and Immunology (Humana Press Inc). 2019;**57**:456-466

[17] Bratten JR, Spanier J, Jones MP. Lactulose breath testing does not discriminate patients with irritable bowel syndrome from healthy controls. American Journal of Gastroenterology. 2008;**103**(4):958-963. DOI: 10.1111/j.1572-0241.2008.01785.x

[18] Chellapandi P, Bharathi M, Sangavai C, Prathiviraj R. Methanobacterium formicicum as a target rumen methanogen for the development of new methane mitigation interventions: A review Veterinary and Animal Science (Amsterdam: Elsevier B.V.). 2018;**6**:86-94

[19] Sahakian AB, Jee SR, Pimentel M. Methane and the gastrointestinal tract. Digestive Diseases and Sciences (Springer New York, NY, USA). 2010;**55**(8):2135-2143

[20] Triantafyllou K, Chang C, Pimentel M. Methanogens, methane and gastrointestinal motility. Journal of Neurogastroenterology and Motility (Seoul, South Korea: Korean Society of Neurogastroenterology and Motility). 2014;**20**(1):31-40

[21] Park YM, Lee YJ, Hussain Z, Lee YH, Park H. The effects and mechanism of action of methane on ileal motor function. Neurogastroenterology and Motility. 1 Sep 2017;**29**(9):e13088

[22] Kim G et al. Methanobrevibacter smithii is the predominant methanogen in patients with constipation predominant IBS and methane on breath. Digestive Diseases and Sciences. 2012;**57**(12):3213-3218. DOI: 10.1007/s10620-012-2197-1

[23] De Lacy Costello BPJ, Ledochowski M, Ratcliffe NM. The importance of methane breath testing: A review. Journal of Breath Research (Bristol, UK: IOP Publishing). 2013;**7**(4):047001

[24] Plauzolles A et al. Small intestinal bacterial overgrowths and intestinal methanogen overgrowths breath testing in a real-life French cohort. Clinical and Translational Gastroenterology. 2023;**14**(4):e00556. DOI: 10.14309/ctg.0000000000000556

[25] Saad RJ, Chey WD. Breath testing for small intestinal bacterial overgrowth: Maximizing test accuracy. Clinical Gastroenterology and Hepatology. 2014;**12**(12):1964-1972. DOI: 10.1016/j.cgh.2013.09.055

[26] Pimentel M, Kong Y, Park S. IBS subjects with methane on lactulose breath test have lower postprandial serotonin levels than subjects with hydrogen. Digestive Diseases and Sciences (New York, NY, USA: Springer). 2004;**49**(1):84-87

[27] Lecours PB, Marsolais D, Cormier Y, Berberi M, Haché C, Bourdages R, et al. Increased prevalence of Methanosphaera stadtmanae in inflammatory bowel diseases. PLoS One. 3 Feb 2014;**9**(2):e0087734

[28] Coker OO, Wu WKK, Wong SH, Sung JJY, Yu J. Altered gut archaea

composition and interaction with bacteria are associated with colorectal cancer. Gastroenterology. 2020;**159**(4):1459-1470.e5. DOI: 10.1053/j.gastro.2020.06.042

[29] Chaudhary PP, Conway PL, Schlundt J. Methanogens in humans: potentially beneficial or harmful for health. Applied Microbiology and Biotechnology (Springer Verlag). 2018;**102**:3095-3104

[30] Armougom F, Henry M, Vialettes B, Raccah D, Raoult D. Monitoring bacterial community of human gut microbiota reveals an increase in *Lactobacillus* in obese patients and methanogens in anorexic patients. PLoS One. 23 Sep 2009;**4**(9):e07129

[31] Tremlett H, Bauer KC, Appel-Cresswell S, Finlay BB, Waubant E. The gut microbiome in human neurological disease: A review. Annals of Neurology (John Wiley and Sons Inc). 2017;**81**:369-382

[32] de Jonge WJ. The Gut's little brain in control of intestinal immunity. ISRN Gastroenterology. 2013;**2013**:1-17. DOI: 10.1155/2013/630159

[33] Wang Y, Kasper LH. The role of microbiome in central nervous system disorders. Brain, Behavior, and Immunity (Academic Press Inc). 2014;**38**:1-12

[34] Pimentel M, Gunsalus RP, Rao SS, Zhang H. Methanogens in human health and disease. The American Journal of Gastroenterology Supplements. 2012;**1**(1):28-33. DOI: 10.1038/ajgsup.2012.6

[35] Drancourt M et al. Evidence of archaeal methanogens in brain abscess. Clinical Infectious Diseases. 2017;**65**(1):1-5. DOI: 10.1093/cid/cix286

[36] Strandwitz P et al. GABA-modulating bacteria of the human gut microbiota. Nature Microbiology. 2019;**4**(3):396-403. DOI: 10.1038/s41564-018-0307-3

[37] Wang T, van Dijk L, Rijnaarts I, Hermes GDA, de Roos NM, Witteman BJM, et al. Methanogen levels are significantly associated with fecal microbiota composition and alpha diversity in healthy adults and irritable bowel syndrome patients. Microbiology Spectrum. 21 Dec 2022;**10**(6):e02290-22

[38] Fattorusso A, Di Genova L, Dell'isola GB, Mencaroni E, Esposito S. Autism spectrum disorders and the gut microbiota. Nutrients (MDPI AG). 2019;**11**:521-535

[39] Oleskin AV, Shenderov BA. Probiotics and Psychobiotics: The Role of Microbial Neurochemicals. New York LLC: Springer; 2019. DOI: 10.1007/s12602-019-09583-0

[40] Vierbuchen T. Innate Recognition and Inflammasome Activation in Human Myeloid Immune Cells by Methanogenic Archaea. [Dissertation]. Bonn, Germany: University of Bonn; 2018

[41] Choileáin SN, Kleinewietfeld M, Raddassi K, Hafler DA, Ruff WE, Longbrake EE. CXCR3+ T cells in multiple sclerosis correlate with reduced diversity of the gut microbiome. Journal of Translational Autoimmunity. 1 Jan 2020;**3**:100031

[42] Czajkowska A, Szponar B. Short chain fatty acids (SCFA), the products of gut bacteria metabolism and their role in the host. Postępy Higieny i Medycyny Doświadczalnej. 2018;**72**:131-142. DOI: 10.5604/01.3001.0011.6468

[43] Bang C, Weidenbach K, Gutsmann T, Heine H, Schmitz RA. The intestinal archaea *Methanosphaera stadtmanae* and *Methanobrevibacter smithii* activate

human dendritic cells. PLoS One. 10 Jun 2014;**9**(6):e0099411

[44] Bang C, Vierbuchen T, Gutsmann T, Heine H, Schmitz RA. Immunogenic properties of the human gut-associated archaeon *Methanomassiliicoccus luminyensis* and its susceptibility to antimicrobial peptides. PLoS One. 1 Oct 2017;**12**(10):e0185919

[45] Low K, Hwang L, Hua J, Zhu A, Morales W, Pimentel M. A combination of rifaximin and neomycin is most effective in treating irritable bowel syndrome patients with methane on lactulose breath test. Journal of Clinical Gastroenterology. 2010;**44**(8):547-550

[46] Samuel BS, Gordon JI. A humanized gnotobiotic mouse model of host-archaealbacterial mutualism. Proceedings of the National Academy of Sciences of the United States of America. 2006;**103**(26):10011-10016

[47] Gaci N, Borrel G, Tottey W, O'Toole PW, Brugère JF. Archaea and the human gut: New beginning of an old story. World Journal of Gastroenterology (WJG Press). 2014;**20**:16062-16078